Nursing School Thrive Guide

MAUREEN OSUNA, BSN, RN

ISBN-10: 1500956368
ISBN-13: 978-1500956363
www.straightanursingstudent.com

DEDICATION

This book is dedicated to my mom, who always believed I was
capable of accomplishing anything I wanted. She was right.

TABLE OF CONTENTS

ACKNOWLEDGMENTS

This book was made possible by a husband who has plenty of interests of his own and therefore stays out of my hair, exceptional nursing professors of CSU Sacramento, a cat who is only moderately needy, and the best group of ICU nurses and docs one could ever hope to work with. And of course, it would not be possible without you, the nursing student. You are my inspiration and it brings me great joy to help you on this exciting journey. Enjoy!

CHAPTER ONE

BEFORE CLASS STARTS

Congratulations! You've been accepted into the nursing program and now you're a bundle of nerves, excitement and eager anticipation as to what this next chapter in your life will bring. Well I am here to tell you that it can be one of the best times of your life if you plan properly, stay organized and take time to treat yourself well. Maybe you've heard nothing but horror stories about how "nursing school takes over your life" or you'll be "lucky to just pass." To all that, I say PHOOEY! You don't have to let nursing school take up your every waking moment and you can forget about "just passing your courses" right now...with my tips you will not only survive, but you will thrive! Whether you've got three months or three days before class starts, I highly recommend getting your ducks in a row before the you-know-what hits the fan. Yes, nursing school is VERY busy, but you are going to maximize your time by planning ahead and doing a bit of prep work before class starts. So, get on your running shoes and let's get going!

Go Shopping

In addition to buying everything on your school's must-have list (stethoscope, scrubs, etc...), you'll want to do a little shopping and stock up on staple items. These are things you use all the time and won't spoil. We're talking shampoo, soap, deodorant, hair gel, toilet paper, feminine hygiene supplies, non-perishable food items, pet food, cat litter, laundry detergent, printer ink, paper and anything else you don't want to shop for over the next few months. You will have very little time for luxuries like grocery shopping, so get as much done now as you can. Another option is to utilize Amazon's Subscribe & Save program to schedule regular (and discounted) delivery of frequently used items.

Clean Like You've Never Cleaned Before

Trust me when I tell you that you aren't going to have as much time as you'd like to dedicate to keeping your nest beautifully feathered (but you WILL have time to do basic upkeep if you follow my tips coming up in chapter five.) With that said, by starting things off with an immaculate and well-organized home, you set yourself up for a sane start to your semester and a home that can be maintained with minimal effort for the next few months. This means doing ALL the laundry, cleaning out the gunk from under the kitchen sink, organizing your pantry, scrubbing the bathroom... the whole shebang. Clean like it's the first day of spring, and you'll love the feeling of having a tidy home to go with your tidy and well-organized nursing student brain.

Get Rid of Clutter

Now is the perfect time to go through every room in the house and get rid of clutter. Start with the room you'll be using the most, which is your office or whatever room houses your study materials/desk. For some of you, this is a bedroom, a den or even a dining room table. Get this area de-cluttered and functional. If you have trouble getting motivated, set a timer for 10-15 minutes and get rid of as much stuff as you can in that time frame...repeat this over and over until you have an efficient and pristine work area. Continue throughout the rest of the house and you'll love the feeling of having a clutter-free home to come home to at the end of the day.

Plan Your Meals

Clear some space in your freezer and put together some meals you can pop in the oven or the crockpot on busy days. Even if you are cooking for one, you can scale things down and utilize the small aluminum trays or single-serving plastic containers. Really, there's no excuse not to do this very important task. There are a ton of online resources for make-ahead freezer meals, and if you live in a city with a freezer meal service, grab a friend and spend an evening making 30 dinners. On those nights when you have to study or work on a project, you'll be so glad you took this simple step. While your classmates are resorting to microwave pizza, you'll be dining on chicken cacciatore or zesty cheese enchiladas. Sounds good, doesn't it? I can't stress enough how important it is that you take care of yourself during nursing school, and good food is one way to do just that.

Be Boring at Lunch

Plan ahead for some easy on-the-go lunches you can schlep around school or clinical all day. When I say "be boring" I'm suggesting you just come up with three or four variations so you can plan ahead and not have to waste brain cells or time on the "what should I take for lunch tomorrow" question. Easy and healthy lunches/snacks include sandwiches, sliced apples with peanut butter or almond butter, Lara Bars, handfuls of nuts, raw veggies and hummus, hard boiled eggs, grapes...you get the idea. By ensuring you always have something nutritious at hand, you will avoid wasting time and money eating out. Plus, nothing blows an awesome study session like the hungries, so fuel up and keep those brain cells humming along!

Wake up on Time, Every Time

When I was a student I was so paranoid about missing my alarm. What if the power went out, what if my cell phone stopped working, what if there was a zombie apocalypse? Would I get to clinical on time? So, I opened an account with wakeupcalls.net, a wake-up call service that calls you at the time you designate. You can even make it say things like "good morning, beautiful" or "go get 'em, Tiger" to get you pumped for your day. Okay, maybe pumped is too strong a word to use for 4:30am, but you know what I mean.

Automate Your Life

Look ahead at the next few months and put things onto autopilot as much as you can. Schedule appointments in advance, put your bills on auto-pay, sign up for Amazon's Subscribe & Save, and schedule your wake-up calls for the next few months. Basically set things in motion now, so you can pretty much not have to worry about them when you're studying for an exam, perfecting a group project or crafting the world's most eloquent care plan.

Get the Gear You Need

Yes, more shopping! Your school is going to send you a list of things you absolutely have to have for classes and clinical. This will include items such as your stethoscope, a pair of calipers, hemostats and scissors. You'll also want to invest in a good pair of shoes for your clinical days. I highly recommend you get the most comfortable shoes you can afford, but don't go wild...your school will likely dictate that you wear white shoes (I have no idea why, but this seems to be universal), and I can guarantee that you won't want to ever wear them again. Ever. With that said, get a pair that make your feet happy, and preferably a pair that don't have any cloth or canvas so you can clean any gunk off them easily.

I also highly recommend a rolling backpack. Yes, I know they're dorky. But I also know you will be lugging around a lot of books and supplies and it would be nice if you saved your back for things like doing actual nursing. A rolling backpack is a lifesaver...find one with lots of compartments for keeping all your stuff organized and roll that baby around with pride. So, what are you going to stock your oh-so-cool rolling backpack with? I found that the following list of items came in handy on a pretty regular basis:

- Mini stapler
- Mini three-hole punch
- Staple remover
- Pens
- Mechanical pencil with extra lead and erasers
- Calculator
- Pharmacology reference (book or electronic)
- Lab reference (book or electronic)
- Planner/calendar
- Change for the vending machine and copy machine
- Spare phone charger
- Ear buds for your cell phone, iPod, mp3 player

You will also want to spend a little time at the office supply store stocking up on things you'll need to study the *Straight A* way:

- Highlighters (various colors)
- Page tabs and flags
- One Mega-Binder, 4 or 5-inches
- Two 2-inch binders, durable and two different colors
- Page dividers with pockets (get two times the number of classes you have, plus another packet or two for clinical). If you can find page dividers that coincide with the colored paper you're also going to buy, get those!
- Colored paper (one pack is more than enough...share with a friend!)

Start Your Nursing Library

Don't go crazy and buy every nursing reference book out there, but do invest in a few staples you will use again and again throughout your program.

I started out with a medical dictionary that I still absolutely love, Lippincott's *Manual of Nursing Practice* (I used this a ton), a care plan book by Gulanick & Myers, a book titled *Fluids & Electrolytes* by Chernecky that I still find extremely useful today, and another Lippincott book titled *Handbook of Medical-Surgical Nursing*. To make things easy for you, I've linked each of these books on my website. See how easy your life is getting, and you've just started reading this book?

Pharmacology Reference

This can be a book or an online resource/app such as Skyscape. Most of the free online resources/apps lack the amount of detail your coursework will require, so be sure to check them out thoroughly before relying on them in a time of need. Make sure your resource includes the generic and brand names of drugs, drug class, indications, contraindications, side effects, monitoring parameters, dosages and black box warnings.

Lab and Diagnostic Test Reference

This can also be in the form of a book or an online resource/app. The best one I found is by Mosby, I absolutely loved this book and used it a ton.

NCLEX Books

Yes, I know what you're thinking. You're thinking that you're not going to be taking the NCLEX for a loooong time, so why start studying now? The reason is simple. Your nursing instructors are going to be writing NCLEX-style test questions for which there are often four correct answers and one "most correct" answer. You need to get used to these style of questions ASAP or you will be thoroughly hating life for the next couple of years. Whatever resource you choose, make sure it includes rationales for why the correct answers are correct and the wrong answers are wrong...this is an invaluable way to study! I found the ones by Saunders and Mosby to be the best, and I tried a lot of different books, so trust me on this one.

If you are a little afraid of NCLEX style questions, the book *Test Success* breaks down how to approach them. Check it out and relieve a load of test anxiety, I guarantee it! Another great book is called *Fundamentals Success*. It also has NCLEX questions and includes a solid review of nursing fundamentals.

And last, but not least, I have to mention all the *Made Incredibly Easy* books. These are absolutely fabulous, very readable and they really make things easy to understand. Plus, they are very visual if you are inclined to that sort of thing. They even publish a magazine you might actually set time aside to read.

Okay, so now that you've cleaned, de-cluttered, shopped, cooked and automated you are finally ready to get down to the nitty gritty of getting organized for school. Ready? Let's do this.

CHAPTER TWO

GETTING ORGANIZED

The Binder Situation

Gone are the days of shlepping around a binder for each class. If you did that in nursing school your whole rolling backpack would just be binders, and you've got to save room for books, more books and your ration of emergency snacks. With the *Straight A* system, you will only need three binders, and you will only need to carry one binder with you at any given time. Yes, you heard that correctly. This magical, amazing binder will contain everything you currently need to absolutely, positively kick some nursing school $@&! The three binders you will need are a daily binder, a Mega Binder and a clinical binder.

Three Binders
Daily Binder
Mega Binder
Clinical Binder

that's it!

If you followed the instructions in chapter one, you treated yourself to a lovely two-inch binder of the heavy-duty variety along with some page dividers and page tabs/flags. Set up your daily binder by labeling each page divider with the name of each class. Toss some page tabs/flags in the front pocket and you're good to go. This binder will contain your notes for each class for the section you are currently studying. Once you take the exam for that section, you move those notes to the Mega Binder. "But wait," you are saying, "those PowerPoint printouts my teacher uses are 20 pages long...I can't fit all those in a two-inch binder!" You're right, you can't. And you also can't thrive in nursing school by relying on slide handouts, so get that out of your head right now. Trust me.

So what is Mega Binder, you ask? Mega Binder is what you will use to archive your paperwork once each unit or module is complete. You will set up your Mega Binder the same way you did your daily binder, with a page divider for each class. You won't need tabs and flags here, since the pages will already be tabbed as needed when they move into the Mega Binder. Don't be afraid to go big here...a four or five-inch binder is hefty, but you won't be carrying it around anywhere (except maaaaybe to study for finals), so it's all good. As you complete a unit (also known as "take a test"), you'll move that material over from your daily binder to the Mega Binder...note that Mega Binder is capitalized. It deserves our respect.

The clinical binder is the one you will use to organize your care plans, clinical paperwork, check-off lists and clinical projects. One suggested way to organize this information is to have page dividers labeled as care plans, clinical paperwork, projects and misc. Within the care plans section, use your nifty page tabs to denote each week. Use the "misc" section for stuff that doesn't fit anywhere else such as reference material, phone numbers of your clinical group members, codes for all the doors on the different units you work on, etc... Now that you have all your binders set up and ready for action, you're ready to start tackling the huge amount of paperwork that will be bombarding you as the semester begins.

The Syllabus Situation
This next step may have to wait until class actually starts, but if your instructors send out your syllabi early, then you can get started geeking out right away. As soon as you get your syllabus from each class, assign it a color from your pack of color-coded paper (you did go shopping, didn't you?) Photocopy or print each syllabus onto colored paper, staple them ALL together and voila...you've got a Mega Syllabus that you will carry with you everywhere. Except maybe the shower...don't take your syllabus into the shower. Now, in a perfect world, your colors coincide with the colors of your page dividers in your daily binder. If that's the case, you get bonus points for being a tad bit OCD...I foresee a future in the ICU for you ;-)

The To-Do List Situation

As you look through each syllabus you are going to be overwhelmed with all the "to-do" items. Never fear, we are going to make them manageable the *Straight A* way! For this project, you'll need a spreadsheet program such as Excel or Numbers...I'm guessing Google docs would also work, though I haven't tried it so don't quote me on that. Start a spreadsheet with the headers TASK, DUE DATE, CLASS and DONE.

Next, start going through each syllabus and type in each and every task you have to do. Even if it's not an assignment, but something like "turn in immunization form" or "select topic for patient education project"... whatever it is, give it a line in your spreadsheet. You will also put the date the task is due and what class it's for. Don't worry about putting things in order as you go, that's what the "sort" feature is for. Once you're finished putting everything in for every single class, sort them by date and TaDa! Now you have a Master Schedule (you thought I was going to call it Mega Schedule, didn't you?). Print this bad boy out and put it in your calendar or daily binder. This schedule will be your holy grail, your bible, your go-to, your everything. And it feels really really really good to check things off this list. Like ridiculously good. You'll see.

The Planner/Calendar Situation

Yes, I know we live in a digital world, but I am a paper girl. To thrive in nursing school I highly recommend using a paper calendar/planner. Not only is it not prone to crashes or batteries that suddenly decide to wimp out on you, but it's also easy to jot things down on-the-go, make lists, write notes and reminders all in one easy-to-access place. I think it's a good idea to supplement your planner with a digital version, but my digital version only included actual appointments, class-times and exam dates. For all the million little tasks and reminders, I wholeheartedly believe you need an actual, physical paper calendar.

With that said, I have designed a planner geared specifically for nursing students (though to be honest it's rather girly...I do plan to make a more unisex version at some point.) Basically, it is the planner I wish I'd had when I was a student. Each week covers two pages, with the area on the left fully devoted to list-making and keeping track of assignments due that week. The right side is your calendar page for scheduling everything you need to do. As an added bonus, each page of the weekly spread has a nursing fact across the top, so you get a little extra knowledge while you plan your week. And, since I am a firm believer in taking good care of ourselves, there's also space for keeping track of your hydration, logging fruit & veggie consumption (aim for nine a day!) and meal or exercise planning. Now that's what I call absolutely nifty! If you prefer something more unisex, I can highly recommend the Uncalendar (available at www.uncalendar.com) which is also great for list-making and keeping things on schedule (and is what I actually used when I was in school, before I developed The Best Planner Ever.) If you're interested in purchasing the *Straight A* Nursing Student planner, visit the website for details at www.straightanursingstudent.com.

Since we're on the topic of planning, I must say a word or two here about flexibility. Nurses must absolutely be flexible when on the job, so it stands to reason that we have to be flexible in school, too. Your schedule will change, things will get moved around and all I have to say is "just go with it." Use a pencil for all things planner related and try not to get too upset when things get tweaked at the last minute. Consider it training for the job and you'll be fine!

CHAPTER THREE

WHAT TYPES OF CLASSES WILL I TAKE?

There are a few different types of classes you'll be taking in nursing school. Hopefully this gives you an idea of what to expect.

Theory Classes

Theory classes are lecture-based courses that cover topics such as professionalism, history of nursing, leadership, research and nursing theories. While it might seem like these courses would be the "easy" ones, they are usually quite tricky for students to master. Maybe it's because most of us gravitate toward the clinical application type courses or because the amount of content to be covered is actually quite immense. Either way, these are not classes you want to take lightly. Research is especially tricky and leadership courses often involve a lot of writing and group projects. And yes, there is a tendency for students to feel like theory-style classes are a waste of time. While you may be all hot and heavy to learn about cardiogenic shock, don't forget that these theory classes provide the framework for nursing as a profession and the backbone for everything you do. Now, go sit and enjoy your three-hour lecture on nursing theorists, the American Red Cross and the Crimean War.

Skills Lab

Skills lab is the class that makes people cry. It's true. There is a ton of information to learn for skills lab. An absolute ton. On top of that you have scary-as-heck professors watching you like hungry hawks, instructors calling you out on the teeniest and tiniest of mistakes, and skills check-offs that can get you booted from the program faster than you can perform hand hygiene.

This is the class where you learn how to do nursey stuff. You'll start with the basics such as taking vital signs and progress to giving injections, starting IVs, inserting Foley catheters, performing fetal monitoring, and changing dressings. It's the most hands-on of all your classes and can be really fun if you can just relax and enjoy it. You will need to study your tail off for this class though as it typically covers topics known as "nursing fundamentals," which is basically how to do absolutely everything step by microscopic step. Take a peek at your fundamentals book and you'll see what I mean.

Simulation

Simulation is the most fun you ever had while being afraid you might actually wet yourself in the process. It is a very intimidating type of class, but you will soon get somewhat used to it and that's when the party starts. Most schools utilize simulation to allow students the opportunity to put their assessment and critical thinking skills to the test in a safe, supportive and learning environment (in other words, you get to practice on a mannequin before you go practice on real people...whew!)

In simulation scenarios, your mannequin will breathe, talk, have lung sounds, a heartbeat, and a pulse. He acts pretty much like a real patient except he doesn't have annoying family members and doesn't constantly get on the call light to ask for more pudding (did I just say that?). He will have a monitor so you can watch his vital signs (provided you connect him to the monitor, of course), and there will be someone behind a one-way mirror who is manipulating the mannequin and the entire situation. You will have meds available as well as all the equipment you might need such as an ambu-bag, intubation materials, Foley cath, IV supplies and medications.

Simulation usually starts off with your patient off the monitor, hanging out breathing room air and saying something really vague like, "I don't feel well." You then go in with a few other classmates and do an assessment, intervene, reassess, and so on and so on. This is where you'll want to use your Nursing Process (you paid attention in theory class, right?) and your clinical judgment and critical thinking (you paid attention in Med/Surg class, right?). You'll also be working as a team with your other classmates, so clear communication is key. And don't worry if your patient dies. You're not getting graded on that, it's simply a learning experience. You'll be fine.

Clinical-Based Lectures

These classes are the nuts and bolts of your nursing education. They are your "Big Daddy" classes in that they provide the clinical knowledge you will use to pass your NCLEX, rock it in clinicals and be an awesome nurse on the job. You will spend the majority of your time studying and prepping for these classes and you will love every minute of it. Okay, maybe that's an exaggeration, but you will most likely enjoy these classes more than the others. These classes are typically called something like *Med-Surg, Advanced Med-Surg, OB, Peds, Mental Health* and *Community Health.* They are the courses that have a clinical component to them, meaning you'll also be spending time in the hospital, mental health facility, and out in the community. If you need help with these classes, never fear. I saved most of my notes from nursing school and have made them available on my website. But you're also going to be making your own notes, so don't start thinking you're getting off easy. More on that in a bit.

Clinicals

Clinical refers to the time you spend working for free and learning how to be a nurse in the patient care setting. You'll typically have one to two clinical days each week, and you will spend an inordinate amount of time doing your "clinical prep." This involves going to the hospital the day before your actual clinical day to select the patients you are going to work with. You then go home and do your clinical prep, which includes a whole lot of paperwork and the writing of the dreaded care plan. More on that in chapter seven, *How to Be a Clinical Rockstar.*

For mental health clinical, you'll do your time at some kind of mental health facility and may also spend time doing some kind of outpatient mental health nursing as well. We did both and it made for a very busy semester!

For community health clinical, you'll be working at a community health agency and interacting with people in the...you guessed it...community. The scope of community health is very broad, here are a few examples:

• working for a county in-home health services agency, visiting clients in their homes, conducting interviews and performing assessments

- working at a community health agency to decrease the incidence of disease in a specific population
- working at a shelter to educate residents about healthy behaviors
- working with a school district to help keep high risk students healthy and in school

So now that you know a little bit about what to expect from each type of class, you might be interested in learning how you're going to study for each class. If so, read on!

CHAPTER FOUR

LEARNING STYLES – EMBRACE THEM ALL!

By now in your academic career I can only assume you've taken those quizzes a million times to determine if you're a visual learner, auditory learner, kinetic learner, etc... One of the things you may have noticed about those tests is that rarely is anyone 100 percent in any particular category. So, even though you may skew toward being a visual learner, it doesn't mean it's the only way you can learn. In fact, I'm going to go out on a limb and suggest that your brain is amazing enough to learn in a variety of ways. So with that said, I have good news and more good news. We are going to learn things YOUR way. In fact, we are going to learn things in EVERY way. That's the *Straight A* way and it works. In fact, it works so well you might just surprise yourself. Are you ready?

- Visual Learner: For the visual side of our brains we will be drawing pictures, making diagrams, studying graphics, using color coding and watching videos.
- Verbal Learner: For the verbal side of our brains, we will be talking... mostly to ourselves but sometimes to others.
- Kinetic Learner: For the tactile/kinetic side of our brains we will be doing things, performing tasks, practicing skills.

- Auditory Learner: For the auditory side of our brains we will be listening to lectures (obviously), but also listening to content that has a direct connection to ourselves.
- Logical Learner: For the logical side of our brains we will be categorizing and re-organizing information.
- Social Learner: The social butterfly in all of us will be working in small groups on occasion...emphasis on the word "small." I am not a big fan of large study groups.
- Solitary Learner: The solitary side of us will be working at our own pace while utilizing the tools that work best for us.

We'll talk more about incorporating each of these learning styles in the next chapter when we get down to the nitty-gritty of studying the *Straight A* way.

CHAPTER FIVE

STUDYING THE *STRAIGHT A* WAY

Now that you've got your schedule all planned out and know what you need to do when you need to do it, you can make space in your brain for actually tackling the massive amount of content you need to learn in nursing school.

Studying the *Straight A* way can best be described as an inverted pyramid. At the top of the pyramid you are gaining a general understanding of the topic. As you move through the levels of the pyramid, you will refine your knowledge step-by-step until you get to a place of mastery and this is when you are tested on the material (and when you totally rock that test!) It is a proven technique that works exceptionally well. Here's how:

Skim Chapters, Get A Broad Understanding

Prior to attending class, you are going to skim the chapter(s) to be discussed. Notice I didn't say "read" the chapters...who has time for that? Certainly not you! You will, instead, skim each chapter. Focus on the chapter headers, the first paragraph of each section and pay particular attention to graphics, side bars, call-outs, diagrams, pictures and photographs. These are used in the textbook for a reason, and the reason is that they are Very Very

Important! If there's anything you don't understand initially, consider looking it up online for a quick reference, but be careful not to get bogged down here. You just want to start your brain thinking in the right direction; we'll get more focused later. This is the very first step in the pyramid Congratulations! You are studying the *Straight A* way already and you haven't even been to class!

Attend Lecture

Most of your classes will be taught in lecture format with a large screen in the front of the room showing slides from some kind of presentation program (usually PowerPoint, so that's what we'll call it here). Your instructor will most likely email or post the PowerPoint slides in advance so you can bring them with you to class and use them to study from later on. You have two options

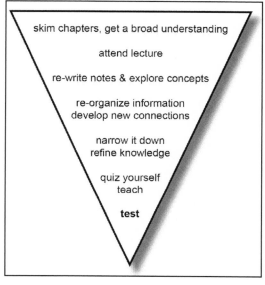

here and you will notice that neither one of them involves printing out the slides and using them to study for the test.

Option 1 is to print out the slides so that you have no more than six per sheet and write your notes directly on the page. Note that if you choose this option you will still be taking things a step further. You will not be using this chaotic, unorganized mess to try and study for the test. Option 2 (and the one I recommend) is to open the PowerPoint presentation and view it in outline mode. You will then copy this outline and paste it into a Word document, meaning it will no longer look like individual slides but like an actual outline. You will then be taking your laptop to class (provided this is allowed), and typing your notes in as the instructor is lecturing. If the instructor does not allow laptops in class, print out your outline with lots of space between the lines so you can write in your notes by hand. Whatever option you choose, you will be leaving class with slides or an outline augmented by your own notes.

Rewrite Notes & Explore Concepts

This is where the good times start to roll. After lecture, you are going to rewrite your notes. Gone are the days of trying to study for an exam off some disjointed PowerPoint slides your instructor lectured on three weeks ago. If you have ever tried to look back at PowerPoint lectures, you will see that it's really just a bunch of bullet points, with no indication of how one concept relates to the next. Take a look at this sample slide from a lecture on diabetic ketoacidosis. Are you going to remember how these concepts relate when you look at this slide and your scribbled notes a month from now?

> ### DKA - Assessment
> -K, Na
>   - cardiac, hypotonic solution
> -Urine Output
> -Blood glucose level (50-70/hr)
> -Serum Osmol
> -Anion Gap

By rewriting your notes soon after the lecture, you will be solidifying those connections and concepts so they stick in your brain. You may think this takes a long time, but it is well worth it! As you rewrite the notes, you are actually studying, plus you are making it super easy to reference these ideas later on. Here's how that slide gets re-written into everyday language so that you can remember how things connect a month (or even years) later:

In DKA, you will watch for fluctuation in electrolyte values since potassium moves into the cell along with the glucose. As you give insulin to "unlock" the cell, the potassium and glucose will enter the cell together, and you can end up with low K levels and cardiac problems. Because of the massive diuresis, you will also need to watch serum Na and serum Osmolality... if serum Na levels rise with all the normal saline you're giving you may need to switch to a hypotonic solution. Along those same lines, you'll keep a close eye on urine output as a way to monitor fluid balance and kidney function. You will also be checking blood glucose levels every hour...you are aiming for them to decrease by 50-70 mg/dL each hour. By keeping an eye on the anion gap, you will know when your patient is ready to transition off the infusion and start on regular sub-q insulin injections.

As you rewrite your notes, write them in a conversational style, as though you were explaining this stuff to a friend. Use examples to help bring concepts to life, and if you're fuzzy on something, augment your lecture with trusted online resources and your text. If you typed notes in class using your outline, then you are a step ahead as now you just go into your document and expand on concepts, fix all the typos you made from typing so fast, format it so it looks uniform and add in graphics as needed. To add in graphics, I used the

Something else I highly recommend is taking the instructor's objectives for each section and writing up notes specific for each objective. Yes, it is extra work, but I found that this helped narrow down what I truly needed to study for the exams.

online references that came with my textbooks, copied and pasted them into my notes. Remember, we are using ALL learning styles, so even if you don't consider yourself a "visual learner," add in some visuals...you'll be glad you did! This is also a great time to incorporate videos into your learning. Many medical device companies post their instructional videos on YouTube, so if you're curious how something works, you can likely find a video that explains it all. I also recommend using a font that doesn't take up a ton of space (arial narrow is great). Print your notes two-sided and now you'll see how a 20-page PowerPoint presentation can fit into your daily binder as a four to five-page document that's highly relevant and usable. You're a genius!

Once your notes are printed, you may want to utilize color coding to help key information pop. For example, I used different colored highlighters to draw attention to things I needed to memorize. All medications were highlighted in green, all sizes of things (Foley catheters, needle gauges, etc...) were orange, all lab values blue, all time intervals were pink. You get the idea.

Reorganize Information
This is where the true studying really begins and is probably one of the best study tips I can offer. By reorganizing information, you make new connections in your brain and develop multiple ways to retrieve data. For example, when studying the muscles in A&P, I reorganized the information and made lists of muscles by where they attached (for instance, all the muscles

that attached at the greater trochanter), and by what they did (all the muscles that laterally rotate the thigh...you get the idea). So, as you are going through your notes, look for ways to categorize and reorganize information. Make lists, charts and graphs. Get creative! For another example, let's say you're taking a pharmacology class. It might be interesting to make lists of drugs that have black box warnings, drugs that increase the heart rate, drugs that cause dangerously low blood pressures, drugs that have an antidote, drugs that don't have an antidote, drugs that can ONLY be mixed with D5W, IV drugs that require a filter, etc...now doesn't that sound fun?

Narrow It Down and Refine Knowledge

As you study, you are going to start storing things in long-term memory (which is exactly where you want it to go.) Let's say you have 10 pages of typed-up notes on taking care of the pediatric cardiovascular patient (and man-oh-man, do those kids have some interesting cardiac defects!). Get out a pencil and a piece of blank paper and jot down notes JUST on the things you still need to study. If you've got something down and totally "get it", you can leave that information out or just write down a very simple phrase to help you retrieve it. The idea is that as you go along, more and more information will get relegated to long-term memory as your notes become shorter and shorter. I found it really convenient to just carry around 10 or so of these reference sheets and study the highlights as I got closer to the exam and more and more information was in my long-term memory. Once your topics are down to less than one page each, consider yourself "all studied up!" It is now time to move on to the next stage.

Quiz Yourself and Teach It

To further help you get a solid grasp on the information you need to rock the heck out of nursing school you will be quizzing yourself and teaching others. To quiz yourself, you can do one of two things (or both). The first way I like to quiz myself is by making audio files that I can listen to on the run. Now, these aren't your typical audio files. These are files that are basically Q&A exercises so that you can quiz yourself, hear information and talk out loud (remember all those learning styles we're hitting on, don't you?). To do this method, you'll need some kind of recording device. I use GarageBand on my Mac and I am sure there are loads of other ways to go about it. Then, just go through your notes and record yourself asking quiz questions. Be sure to PAUSE long enough in between the question and the answer to give yourself time to answer it when you're listening later on. For example, it might go like this:

"How do you calculate the anion gap in DKA?"
PAUSE
"Add sodium and potassium, then subtract chloride and
bicarb."

During that pause is when you will answer it out loud as you are listening to the recording. Got it? I can't stress enough how awesome this technique is! I used it for most of my classes, even the theory ones. Once I started using this technique, my house got clean, I started going for walks and runs, the laundry got washed and the errands were done. Using these audio quiz files freed me from my desk and allowed me to utilize a different part of my brain (and a different learning style) while getting things done around the house! I felt like a more balanced person and the stress melted away as I was able to keep things tidy and in order.

Another way you can quiz yourself is by making flashcards. Again, these aren't your mamma's flashcards. We are going to utilize technology and create flashcards SUPER FAST that we can easily tote anywhere and use anytime we have a few spare minutes. This technique requires a smart phone, namely an iPhone or Android. To make these amazing flashcards, you just create a spreadsheet in Google Docs, follow the directions at the gFlash website (see the Appendix for the URL) and voila...you have flashcards you can easily tote around with no worry that they'll go flying all over the place. Please note that gFlash currently (as of July 12, 2014) does not work with the updated version of Google Sheets, so be sure you're using the older version for now. Besides gFlash, there are a number of other flashcard programs out there such as CueCard, Anki, and Rememberize. I haven't used any of these, but if you just Google it, I'm sure you'll find something wonderful and easy to use. I'm not sure about the other programs, but with gFlash you can also easily share your flashcard sets with friends, which is sure to gain you popularity points among your classmates.

The third way you are going to quiz yourself is by doing loads and loads of NCLEX practice questions. Buy a book, buy an app, or look them up online. As mentioned before, the best resources will have the rationales for the answers and the questions will be organized by body system. You may even get to a point where you actually enjoy doing the questions, they can actually be kind of fun in a twisted, nerdy sort of way.

In addition to quizzing yourself, you are also going to teach the material. You can do this by hosting a study session (a SMALL one) or simply by making an audio recording of yourself explaining key concepts. Again, you can share these audio files with others, or just use them yourself as a way to augment your studying. For example, when I was learning all the psychiatric drugs, I wrote little stories about each class of drugs using key words that described the side effects. I then recorded an audio file of myself reading these short little stories and when it came time to take the test, all I had to do was recall a silly little story in order to remember that atypical antidepressants cause dizziness and a dry mouth. As an example, below is the little story I made up for that...you'll love it (maybe).

> *The **atypical** girl was **heartbroken** and **depressed** after her boyfriend left her. She **couldn't eat, she couldn't sleep**. She was so upset that she felt **sick to her stomach** all the time, causing horrible **diarrhea**. She was very **confused** about why her boyfriend would leave her, but the truth was, her boyfriend left because of her **low libido**...it seems she always "had a **headache**." She wanted to please her boyfriend, but every time she thought about sex she got **nervous, felt dizzy** and broke out into a **sweat**. Her **hands would shake** so bad that she couldn't even hold a glass of water and take a drink... talk about having a **dry mouth**!*

Test

Now that you've gone through every layer of the pyramid, you are ready to take that test and show it who's boss! But first, you need a solid test-taking strategy to help reduce anxiety so you can relax and let all that information flow freely from that beautiful brain of yours. I highly highly recommend getting a good night's sleep the night before your exam and then AVOID STUDYING the morning of your test. You will see your classmates cramming at the last minute and you will be soooo tempted to jump in there and cram right along with them. Don't do it! Instead of getting caught up in the pre-test cram-a-thon frenzy, I would bring along a set of earbuds and listen to a playlist I created specifically for test days. I loaded it with relaxing and peaceful music, and instead just chilled out while everyone around me freaked out, got their blood pressure up, amped their anxiety and generally had a pretty miserable time. It's a strategy that worked well for me and I know it will work well for you, too.

Another great strategy to utilize is to carefully track your grades. I used an iPhone app that allowed me to input my grades along with how they were weighted. It enabled me to know that for my A&P final I didn't even have to show up in order to get an A for the class (I still took the test...I'm not one to back down from a challenge!). Knowing what grade you need can really help focus your studying or get you to relax a bit, whatever the case may be.

CHAPTER SIX

WOULD YOU LIKE A LATTE WITH THAT?

Now we get to the Most Useful Thing you can learn from this book. It's called LATTE and it's a systematic way to zero in on what you need to focus on in order to care for your patient (both in clinical and on your exams).

LATTE was born in my first semester of nursing school when I was absolutely overwhelmed with all the available data out there. Our instructor would give us case studies to work on and I swear it was like solving a medical mystery each and every time. For example, she'd say, "you have a 43-year old female with liver disease, she's complaining of shortness of breath and her AST/ALT are elevated." We'd then go on these massive data quests to figure out absolutely every single little thing we could about liver disease and sometimes these case studies would be 10 pages long. It took forever and was major overkill. So, one day as I was sitting at my computer working up a case study, I looked over to the ever-present cup of coffee sitting on my desk and I had an idea.

What if I could really focus my brainpower on what I actually need to focus on? What if I had a systematic way to approach each case so that my brain wouldn't go wondering off on wild tangents? What if I had a simple method that worked every single time and ensured I studied the most important information I need for this topic? And that, my friends, is how LATTE was born.

L = LOOK

L stands for "How will your patient LOOK?" In other words, what are their presenting signs/symptoms and what are their chief complaints? What will you see, hear (and even smell) when you walk into the room? For example, with our liver failure patient you'll see jaundiced skin, a distended abdomen, confusion and poor coordination. Your patient will tell you they are short of breath and will probably have pale or grey-colored stool. Maybe they'll be scratching and complaining that they itch all over. For your exams, you'll need to know the classic presenting signs/symptoms for whatever disorder you're studying, so this is where the L comes in.

A = ASSESS

A stands for "How will you ASSESS the patient?" The first step in the nursing process is the most important one you can do. Assess assess and assess! Nurses are constantly assessing their patients, sizing things up with every interaction. I feel sorry for kids who have nurses for parents...they're not getting away with anything! But, I digress. In the case of our liver patient, you'll conduct neuro assessments, check for bleeding at all puncture sites, monitor for increased edema, keep an eye on urine output and so on and so on. With absolutely every interaction with your patient you will be assessing her. She may think you're just chatting her up, but really you're checking to see if she's oriented, making sense, slurring words, having a psychotic break. You'll be checking to see if she can breathe, if she's in pain, how her skin looks, and so on and so forth. Don't discount those interactions with patients just because they're not part of your official "head-to-toe" assessment. You are constantly assessing your patient!

T = TESTS

The first T stands for "What TESTS will be ordered?" Though nurses don't write the orders, you'd be surprised how often you will make recommendations that the physician agrees with. In addition, making recommendations is the "R" in the SBAR communication format (more on that later). By knowing what tests will be ordered, you can anticipate what needs to be done in preparation. Will your patient need to fast, do you need a central line, do you need to coordinate with other members of the team such as respiratory therapists, is your patient going to be "traveling" (leaving the unit and going to CT-scan or MRI, for example). And lastly, knowing what tests are typically ordered cues you in to what test results you'll go searching for in your chart as you follow up from day-to-day and shift-to-shift.

T = TREATMENT

The second T stands for "How will this condition be TREATED?" This is where all your nursing interventions come into play as well as the treatments the physician will order (meds, dialysis, dietary restrictions, etc...) In the case of our liver patient, you'll treat her with things like lactulose (a drug that binds up ammonia), paracentesis to decrease abdominal distension, platelet administration and dextrose.

E = EDUCATE

The E stands for "How will you EDUCATE the patient and the family?" Remember that a key role nurses play is educator. We are constantly teaching our patients and families (whether they listen or heed our advice is something else entirely.) In our liver patient's case, we'll teach about the need for restraints, why we're checking their blood sugar so often, why they're bleeding from their IV sites, how to prevent future complications and the list goes on.

So there you have it. A caffeine-inspired way to streamline your thinking and help you zero in on the absolute most vital information you need to take excellent care of your patients and pass your exams with flying colors. I have put LATTE to the test with a variety of patient scenarios/conditions and it works every single time. Give it a try...I think you'll agree.

CHAPTER SEVEN

BE A CLINICAL ROCKSTAR

All the book smarts in the world aren't worth a darn if you're a dud in clinicals. Your clinical rotation will put your clinical thinking, time management, prioritization and organizational savvy to the test. It will give you opportunities to showcase your compassion, patience and communication skills. Your clinical rotations are all about putting what you've learned at school into real-world application. It will be one of those things you likely dread and enjoy at the same time. Hopefully with my tips, the enjoyment will outweigh any negative emotions brought on by stress or worry. Want to be a clinical rockstar? Here's how you do it.

Pre-Clinical Prep

In most cases, you will be going to the hospital the day before your rotation to select a patient or two to work with. You'll want to choose patients who are not going to be discharged within the next 24 hours and whose needs match your clinical objectives. For example, if you need to practice wet-to-dry dressings, choose a patient with wound care orders. If you need to practice injections, choose a patient who will be receiving their flu or pneumonia vaccines the next day. Try to get a variety of diagnoses so that you're not always taking care of the COPD/pneumonia crowd. Some other basic medical diagnoses you'll see on a Med/Surg unit are diabetic ketoacidosis, sepsis, UTI, decreased level of consciousness (or altered mental status), ischemic or hemorrhagic stroke, respiratory failure, renal failure, cellulitis, bowel obstruction, chest pain, peripheral vascular disease and surgeries of all shapes and sizes. I always tried to choose patients whose diagnosis matched what we were studying that week, but if that's not possible, go for the most interesting cases you can find.

Writing Your Care Plan

Writing up your care plan is probably the most dreaded activity in nursing school, especially in first semester when you are looking up absolutely every little thing. Your clinical instructors will have varying requirements for how they want your care plans written up, but they generally involve making a list of nursing diagnoses and your answer to the most often asked question in nursing, "What are you going to do about it?"

First, we must answer the question, "what exactly is a nursing diagnosis and how does that differ from a medical diagnosis?" This can be a tricky concept for many students to master and one of the most frustrating. Nurses are not licensed to diagnose medical conditions. That's what the physician does when she decides, "Hey, you have congestive heart failure." So while medical diagnoses define the disease or condition a patient has, the nursing diagnoses describe the patient's *response to that diagnosis*. Yes, I know it's muddy. Let's clear things up a bit.

Let's say your physician friend diagnoses your patient with congestive heart failure. One of the problems that patients with heart failure have is edema, often seen as swollen legs and feet. So, your nursing diagnosis for this problem is going to be "fluid imbalance related to congestive heart failure as evidenced by edema on lower extremities." The edema is the patient's response to the congestive heart failure. Get it? Let's do another one.

Your physician friend diagnoses your patient with AIDS, which is causing a whole host of problems. One of those problems is reflected in the nursing diagnosis "risk for imbalanced nutrition: less than body requirements." This is basically a fancy-pants way of saying your patient is at risk for becoming malnourished due to the decreased appetite that comes along with AIDS. See how the nursing diagnoses deals with the patient's response to the disease? Let's do one more.

Your physician pal has also diagnosed your poor patient with liver failure. One of the hallmarks of liver failure is hepatic encephalopathy, which is caused by a buildup of ammonia in the blood. These waste products affect neurological functioning so your nursing diagnosis could be "alteration in mental status related to hepatic encephalopathy as evidenced by ammonia level of 200." Again, the alteration in mental status is the body's response to hepatic encephalopathy.

I hope this helps make the distinction more clear. What can be HIGHLY frustrating for nursing students is that even though we aren't allowed to actually diagnose our patients medically, we still have to have a pretty good idea of what that diagnosis would be so we can respond appropriately. For example, let's say your patient comes in to the ED with an ammonia level of 200 and a distended abdomen. It's super helpful to know he likely has liver failure so you can anticipate what interventions and tests you are going to be performing. But maybe that's just one of my pet peeves? It's possible. I have a lot of pet peeves.

Components of a Nursing Diagnosis

Now that you understand the difference between making a medical diagnosis and a nursing diagnosis, you'll want to get super savvy at writing them so they relate appropriately to your patient. The deal with nursing diagnoses is that you can have one of two types: a potential diagnosis or a definitive diagnosis. The potential diagnosis is something your patient is at risk for, but doesn't necessarily have at this time. This type of diagnosis will always starts with the words "risk for" or "potential." A definitive diagnosis describes something your patient actually does have and always includes the phrase "as evidenced by." In other words, your patient either has a problem or is at risk for having a problem. If he has a problem, you are going to write a definitive diagnosis and must state what the evidence for this is, meaning you're not just making stuff up. You have evidence, proof, or data that they do indeed have this particular problem. This can be information from the chart, something you see on your assessment or even something the patient says. This will become more clear as we do a little practice. For starters, the two types are set up like this:

POTENTIAL DIAGNOSIS
Risk for NURSING DIAGNOSIS
related to (or secondary to) PATIENT'S ISSUE

Example: Risk for PAIN related to HYSTERECTOMY.

DEFINITIVE DIAGNOSIS
NURSING DIAGNOSIS related to (or secondary to)
PATIENT'S ISSUE as evidenced by DATA OBTAINED
FROM ASSESSMENT OR CHART.

Example: PAIN related to HYSTERECTOMY as evidenced by
PATIENT RATING PAIN 7 OUT OF 10.

For example, let's say your 23-year-old patient has had a colectomy with placement of an ileostomy. A few *potential* nursing diagnoses you will use for your care plan are:

• Risk for infection secondary to surgical procedure
• Risk for fluid imbalance secondary to high ileostomy output
• Risk for impaired gas exchange related to pain at surgical site

And a few *definitive* diagnoses you could use are:

• Ineffective coping related to change in body image as evidenced by patient crying and saying, "I'll never go to the beach again."
• Altered nutrition: less than body requirements related to change in dietary requirements as evidenced by patient eating 25% of meals
• Pain secondary to surgery as evidenced by patient rating pain 7 on a 0-to-10 pain scale

The governing board for actual, approved nursing diagnoses is called NANDA, and they are the ones who come up with all this convoluted language to convey your patient's problems. Don't worry, the language gets easier the more you use it. Your professor will require that you use only NANDA-approved diagnoses in your clinical prep. They may sound strange at first, but once you get the hang of them, they'll make much more sense (notice I didn't say they'd make perfect sense, just much more sense!). Here are a few NANDA diagnoses translated into plain English:

• "Impaired gas exchange" means your patient isn't breathing well.
• "Ineffective airway clearance" means the patient can't cough up her secretions, or something is blocking her airway.
• "Ineffective coping" means your patient hasn't found a healthy way to deal with her situation. Maybe she's crying non-stop, regressing developmentally or even having angry outbursts against the staff.
• "Altered nutrition: more than body requirements" means your

patient eats too much as is overweight.

• "Alteration in hemodynamics" means your patients blood pressure, heart rate and/or cardiac function are out of whack.

• "Bathing self care deficit" means your patient hasn't showered lately.

I highly recommend getting a book of nursing diagnoses and using that as your guide throughout this process. I used one by Gulanick and Myers titled *Nursing Care Plans: Diagnosis, Interventions and Outcomes* that was truly great. Having a book of NANDA diagnoses and care plans for all the different problems your patient could have is a lifesaver in nursing school!

Writing Your Care Plan

Your instructor may require a minimum number of diagnoses for each care plan, and may require a certain number of interventions for each one. The best advice I can give for how many nursing diagnoses to include is to look at the orders, notes and meds to come up with an idea of what your patient's problems are. For example, if you see that the physician has ordered pain medicine, then you know pain is a problem or at least a potential problem. At this stage, don't worry about writing out the problems in the somewhat strange language of NANDA, just list them in language you can easily understand (infection, not eating enough, hates her body, dehydration, writhing in pain etc...). Then, consult your list of meds and all the interventions ordered by the physician to get an idea of your "to-do list". For this patient your to-do list may look something like this:

- Cefazolin 1gm IV q 4 hours
- Normal Saline at 75 ml an hour
- Protonix 40 mg PO q day
- Norco 5/325 PO q 6 hours prn mild pain
- Morphine 1 mg IV q 4 hours prn moderate pain
- Morphine 2 mg IV q 4 hours prn severe pain
- Lovenox 40mg SQ daily
- SCDS when in bed
- Ambulate three times a day
- Use incentive spirometer 10x/hr while awake

As you go through each of your problems you will write them as nursing diagnoses and make a list of interventions for each one. As you list an intervention, you are going to cross that item off your "to-do" list. In fact, many of your interventions will come from this list! How cool is that? The idea is that you want to show your clinical instructor that you understand the rational for each med and intervention ordered by the physician. In addition, you will add nursey interventions that don't require an order...things like monitoring her temp, listening to her lung sounds and bowel sounds, encouraging her to eat, communicating therapeutically, providing education about her new dietary requirements, assessing for pain, instructing her to cough/deep breathe, monitoring lab values, etc... Don't worry, this part will become more clear to you as you begin attending classes.

Let's see how this plays out with one of our nursing diagnoses for this patient: *Risk for infection secondary to surgical procedure*. Our interventions might be to:

- Monitor surgical site for signs of infection: redness, warmth, and purulent drainage
- Monitor vital signs for fever, tachycardia, hypotension
- Monitor WBC count
- Listen to lung sounds
- Encourage coughing and deep breathing using the incentive spirometer
- Ambulate TID to encourage deep breathing and lung expansion
- Administer prophylactic antibiotics as ordered
- Administer pain medication as needed to enable patient to take deep breaths

See how this works? If you're just starting out you may not yet understand how these interventions prevent infection. Don't worry about that now, you'll get there soon enough!

There's one more step in your nursing care plan and that is the desired patient outcome from each of your interventions. Let's go back to our "risk for infection" nursing diagnosis. Part of the nursing process is assessment, so after you intervene (also known as "doing nursey stuff") you are going to reassess your patient to see if your intervention worked. So, our desired outcomes might look something like this:

- Wound edges approximated, without redness, swelling, warmth or purulent drainage
- HR < 100 bpm, RR < 20 per minute, blood pressure > 100 systolic, WBC count < 11
- Lung sounds clear with no signs of atelectasis or consolidation

• Patient will ambulate 100 feet three times a day
• Patient will report pain level < 3

The thing with your patient outcomes is that they have to be measurable. You can't just say your patient is going to "walk the halls." You have to say how often and how far they'll walk as in "pt will ambulate 100 feet three times a day." Otherwise, you have no way of definitively knowing if your intervention actually helped your patient meet a goal.

In addition to writing up your nursing diagnoses, interventions and outcomes you will also need to write up your meds. Different instructors have different requirements for this. Some instructors (the clearly diabolical ones) will require that you write these out by hand so that you can't copy and paste from a word processing program from week to week. Others will be fine with using a computer provided you list all the necessary information for each medication. You will need to list the medication name, dosage, route, frequency, why they're getting it, indications, contraindications, mechanism of action, side effects, monitoring parameters, black box warnings (if any), and how you will evaluate its effectiveness. Now, this may seem like no big deal, until you realize a lot of patients are on a LOT of meds. I had one patient who was taking 48 meds every day. I was a little cranky on that one, especially when she refused half of them!

As for the remainder of your clinical prep and care plan, your clinical instructor will have varying requirements and formats. Some will require you to show your schedule for the day indicating when you will perform various interventions and assessments. You may need to write narrative notes and include etiology and pathophysiology of the admitting diagnosis. The main idea with this whole process is to know what you are going to be doing, why you are doing it and how you are going to measure its effectiveness. Once you've done all that, you're ready to show up at clinical and blow everyone away with your awesomeness.

Concept Maps

Concept mapping is becoming a more popular way of doing care plans that shows how all your patient's problems and interventions relate. You will love this method if you are a visual or kinetic learner. It also classifies as "reorganizing information," so it's a super helpful way to create new connections and classify information in that busy busy brain of yours. It's like doing a really fun and super-nerdy puzzle, so if you're into that sort of thing, you'll be totally in your element.

With a concept map, you will show how all your medical diagnoses, conditions, meds and lab results tie together to create an interconnected web that represents your patient at this time. Your clinical professor will have his or her own requirements for your maps, but I will explain how I did mine to at least give you an idea of how you will think through this fun and sometimes complicated process.

I started all my maps by writing the patient's medical diagnoses on a large piece of paper. Let's say your patient has HIV, liver disease and bipolar disorder. Your concept map will start with these three items spaced evenly throughout the page. To differentiate the various elements of your map, use colored pencils or shapes (I used shapes because I erased things so much…diagnoses were bordered with a rectangle, conditions with a puffy cloud shape, meds with a starburst shape and labs with an oval.) Again, your professor may have specific requirements for this, or s/he may want to see how your brain works. Find what works for you and stick with it.

Next you'll want to look through your clinical prep and see what all the patient's conditions and manifestations are. I think of these as the sign and symptoms of his diagnosis. For example, one of the symptoms of HIV infection is fatigue, and he may also have jaundice related to his liver disease. This is when things all start to connect. So, go ahead and write all his conditions and manifestations more or less near the related diagnosis and draw arrows to show how each one connects to the diagnosis that causes it. Note that sometimes a sign or symptom can have more than one cause so draw your arrows accordingly. In this example, both the patient's HIV and his liver disease will contribute to fatigue. See how everything is starting to interconnect?

Now you'll want to go through and look at all his meds. He will be taking each med for a specific reason, so go ahead and write out his meds next to the diagnosis they relate to. Again, use your arrows to indicate which diagnosis requires the use of each med.

And don't forget your lab results. Your patient will likely have a number of abnormal labs, and each of these can be caused by a medical diagnosis, a condition/manifestation or a medication. For example, your patient is taking Trileptal for his bipolar disorder. As you research this medication, you notice it can cause hypocalcemia. Low and behold, your patient's calcium level is low. You will want to place hypocalcemia on the map near your Trileptal, but keep an eye out for other things that can cause this condition. Again, patient's often have multiple contributing factors for the problems they face.

Once you have gone through this process for all your patient's diagnoses, meds, labs and conditions/manifestations, you will have an interconnecting map with arrows and shapes or colors all over the place. Note that many items will have multiple arrows leading to it or branching off from it. For example, this patient has many reasons he would feel fatigue: HIV and its resulting anemia, the meds for HIV, liver disease, bipolar disorder, the depression caused by bipolar disorder and the meds used to treat bipolar disorder. See how it all relates? Check the *Straight A* website for an example.

At Clinical

Either you love clinical or you hate it. I loved it, though I wouldn't say I didn't dread it each and every time. Maybe it had something to do with my scary-as-heck first semester clinical professor or maybe it was just that it was always difficult adjusting to a new unit, new people, new routines and new personalities.

Now, a word or two about clinical instructors. They basically come in one of two types: scary and not scary. Lucky for me, I got the scary type my first semester. An ex-military RN, Professor Rose set exceptionally high standards for her students, demanded their very best and kept us on our toes every single second. Because of this, I developed excellent habits and set a standard of practice for myself that I always think of as stemming from my beloved Professor Rose. One of the best tidbits of advice she ever gave me was simply to "be accurate and be thorough." To this day, when I go through my assessments and charting I always think of these words. If I haven't met Professor Rose's standards for accuracy and thoroughness, I go back and double-check. It's good advice, you should take it.

And then there are the nurses you're working with. Let's face it, Nurses aren't always super friendly when the students show up on the unit, especially if they don't have a choice in the matter. Yes, it is more work (usually) to supervise a student, but it can even out overall if you are a clinical rockstar. Here's my best advice on how to make a fabulous impression on nurses and patients alike. For the record, I love working with students and try to go out of my way to make them feel welcome. When you are a working RN, I encourage you to do the same. It's our way of paying back all the nurses who worked with us when we were in clinical and a way of fostering support and mentorship in the profession.

1) Show up prepared. This goes without saying, but you'd be surprised how often someone is missing a pen, or a stethoscope, or whatever. Whenever I need that one little thing, I always love it when a nearby student whips it out…be it a pair of scissors, an alcohol swab, an end cap or a hemostat. Along the lines of showing up prepared, put some thought into your care plan even if your professor goes easy on you in this regard. It will be glaringly obvious if you show up and don't know what's going on with your patient.

2) Communicate with your RN at the beginning of the shift and let him or her know what you can do unsupervised vs. supervised. If it's first semester and you're all about the ADLs, introduce yourself to the nurses aids and let them know you'd like them to leave your patient's baths and whatnot to you (they'll love the extra help!)

3) Speaking of nurses aids, these angels are seriously your best friends on the floor. Help them out whenever you can and say "thank-you" whenever they do something for you. When you are juggling four to five patients, you will want to hug them at the end of each and every shift. I promise.

4) Make yourself useful. If you've been signed off on a certain skill such as wet-to-dry dressing changes, let your RN know you'd be happy to do additional dressing changes, even for his/her other patients Or, do a few of his other patient's blood sugars for them…something…anything to show everyone how much you appreciate the extra time and effort.

5) Go the extra mile with your patients. Often you'll have just a couple of patients, and while it can seem like you are juggling a lot in the beginning, you may find yourself with some extra time to do those little extras that nurses wish they had time for (but rarely do). I remember one time I gave my patient a foot massage and she about died of happiness. Honestly, it was first semester and I wasn't doing much yet at that point so it was nice to feel useful. I call this the TLC aspect of nursing. Do it while you can!

6) Get in there and practice your skills. Sadly, you may only get to do one Foley insertion the whole time you're in school (most are put in while the patient is in the ED or the OR). Let both your RN and the charge nurse know what skills you'd like to practice. I guarantee you that any RN will jump at the chance to have a student take care of something on their "to-do" list. To ensure the nurse doesn't have to take time out to supervise, ask your professor to come to the floor. Chances are you need to be signed off anyway.

This reminds me of a day when I somehow ended up with two students. One was a student I was precepting for 240 hours and the other was a student that was just there for the day. I split their assignment and had each one take a patient. On top of that, I tried to find things for them to do, since I vividly remember being a student and loving the opportunity to do absolutely anything. Another nurse asked if anyone would care to get her tube feeding set started and my precepted student jumped at the request. The other student, sitting at the nurse's station, indicated she wasn't missing out on anything by not performing this simple task. My opinion of her plummeted right then and there. As students, get up off your tush and offer to help with a smile any and every time it is asked. You never know what you might learn or who you might impress.

7) Do not sit at the nurse's station when there is work to be done. Do not sit. Period.

8) In regards to your assessments and documentation, it can seem overwhelming but really it boils down to those two things that have stuck with me ever since Professor Rose advised me in first semester: "Be accurate and be thorough." Was your head-to-toe accurate? Did you really listen to all four quadrants? If not, go back and do it again. You may find that initially you go back several times to assess "those little things" you forgot the first time around. Don't worry, it gets easier!

9) Never, under any circumstances say, "That's now how they do it at XYZ Hospital." No one cares. Act like you think this unit and hospital are the greatest things since sliced bread. Different places do things differently and it's valuable to learn a variety of methods.

10) When your clinical instructor or preceptor gives you constructive criticism, don't get defensive, don't get long-winded and don't take it personally. Say "thank-you" and move on.

11) And this goes without saying…be professional (no texting!), show your gratitude and have fun!

Charting

Charting is one of those things you'll be immensely anxious about, and for good reason. It is, after all, a legal document. If you are lucky, the facility where you do your clinical rotations will have a user-friendly electronic medical record, but note that some facilities still use paper charting. Unless you are working at the same facility every semester (which is highly unlikely) expect to learn a new charting system every single semester. Remember what I said about nurses being flexible? This is one of those times.

In regards to your charting, your professor may have you write out a narrative note for your head-to-toe assessment. Though your assessment will likely be covered in some kind of flowsheet, many professors want you to have practice at writing in-depth narratives and the head-to-toe assessment is a great place to start. It can, however, be daunting so I've included a couple of examples for you here. You want to say just enough to convey a picture of the patient, without leaving anything open to interpretation.

Received report, assumed care of patient in coordination with Christina, RN. Found pt asleep and disoriented upon waking, pt talking in his sleep and slow to follow commands. HOB flat. VS stable: Temp 36.1, HR 80, RR 13, BP 126/70, O2 99% on RA, pain 5/10, GCS 13. Unable to assess pupils, pt unwilling or unable to open eyes. Pt able to move all four extremities against resistance with slight weakness noted in all extremities. Skin jaundiced, warm and dry. Cardiac sounds normal, no murmurs, regular rhythm. Radial pulses weak and equal. Unable to palpate pedal pulses due to 3+ edema from feet to knee, doppler used, pulses present. Capillary refill <3 seconds in hands and feet. Diminished breath sounds RLL, LLL; no pulmonary secretions present, no complaints of shortness of breath. Abdomen is soft, distended, non-tender. Bowel sounds active in all four quadrants. Pt is voiding amber-colored urine.

And here's another one, this time for a patient in the ICU:

Received report, assumed care of patient under supervision of Thomas, RN. Pt sedated, intubated, restrained, reaches purposefully for ET tube. Pt opens eyes to voice, follows commands, nods or shakes heads to yes/no questions; nods "yes" when asked about pain, fentanyl gtt titrated, see flowsheet. Pupils equal and sluggish; pt moves all four extremities against resistance. HOB at 30-degrees. VS stable on levophed gtt: Temp 37.2, HR 94, RR 19, BP 116/73, O2 97% on vent settings 55% FiO2, tidal volumes 450, PEEP 8, rate 12, PRVC mode. Size 8.0 ETT in place. Breath sounds course in upper lobes, *diminished in lower lobes, thick secretions present. Skin warm, dry, color typical for race. Cardiac sounds assessed, systolic murmur noted, regular rhythm. Pulses strong and equal in all four extremities, capillary refill <3 seconds in hands and feet. Abdomen, soft, non-distended, non-tender, bowel sounds hypoactive in all four quadrants. Tube feeding in place via OGT at 65 cm, placement verified, residual assessed, within normal limits. Foley catheter in place, draining straw-colored urine. Family at bedside, questions answered, reviewed plan for the day.*

See how each of these narrative notes paints a clear picture of your patient? You will also be writing narrative notes for things that happen throughout the day and your nursey response to it. For example, let's start with an easy one and say your patient is complaining of pain in her left arm, on which she recently had surgery to remove an abscess. Apparently she got into an argument with her cat and lost. Your note might look something like this:

1415: At 1355 pt complaining of pain 8/10 at surgical site. 4 mg morphine given at 1400 per MD orders, left upper extremity elevated with two pillows. Pt now stating pain 4/10. Will continue to monitor and provide comfort measures as needed.

A more complicated situation requires a more in-depth note. This patient is complaining of chest pain…and right at change of shift, too!

1840: At 1830, pt complaining of pain 7/10, located in chest and radiating to left arm and jaw. VS as follows: HR 122, BP 167/98, O2 sat 92% on room air, RR 26. Pt placed on 2L oxygen via nasal cannula; morphine, aspirin and nitroglycerin given by RN per protocol, pt states some relief of pain at 5/10. STAT EKG done, showing ST elevation in leads II, III and avF. Cardiac enzymes drawn per protocol. Physician notified, currently at bedside. VS now HR 113, BP 145/86, O2 sat 97% on 2L, RR 22. Cath lab notified of patient's impending arrival. Will continue to monitor.

Notice what these two sample narrative notes have in common. They describe what the patient's problem is, what you did about it, and the patient's response to your intervention. This is the nursing process in action. Pretty nifty, huh?

Time Management

For the nursing student (and new grads), time management can be one of the trickiest skills to learn. When I first started in the ICU, my preceptor kept having to refocus me as I felt like I was being pulled in multiple directions at once. As a student, I remember being insanely busy even when just taking care of two stable "walky-talky" patients. The reason for this is simply that every single thing you are doing is brand spanking new. In addition, you don't yet have a good solid grasp on how to anticipate your patient's needs and you haven't yet developed a routine. Don't worry, we'll get you there.

From your first day of clinical to your last, you will notice that you are always buzzing in and out of your patient's rooms, like a busy little bee. When you have only two patients, this might be okay, but notice that the nurses working on the floor have a full patient load. That's because they have some mad time management skills, and soon you will, too.

One of the key components to effective time management is clustering your nursing activities. I like to follow what I call the High-Five Rule, where I try to do at least five things each time I enter the patient's room. Examples of activities to cluster are: check vital signs, bring hungry patient a snack, empty Foley bag, get patient up to the chair, change dressing on patient's infected big toe.

If you're working in the ICU, the buzzing bee syndrome can be even more pronounced as these critically ill patients are often very busy. You could cluster the following into a High-Five easily: suction ET tube, check blood sugar, check urine output, reposition patient, provide oral care. See how easy it is? If you can consistently give yourself a High-Five each time you go into you patient's room, your time management will flow smoothly. You got this.

Routines

Let's talk a bit about developing routines. Routines are the cornerstone of effective time management as they help you remember to do important tasks in an organized and efficient manner. As you gain experience, you will have the opportunity to create routines that work well for you and the area where you work. As a general rule, I recommend student nurses develop the following routines right off the bat: Start-of-Shift Routine (SOS), First

Assessment Routine (FAR), "Before Leaving the Patient's Room" Routine (Spot Check), and End-of-Shift Routine (EOS).

The Start-of-Shift (SOS) routine consists of all those things you need to do right away so you can take excellent care of your patients. Here's what I like to do for my SOS:

- Check lab results
- Look at MAR, know which meds I'm giving that day and when
- Look at Kardex or RAND for orders: make a plan for the day
- Write out a quick schedule of meds and planned interventions
- Print an EKG strip for patients that are on telemetry monitoring
- Grab some alcohol swabs and end-caps for my pockets

The First Assessment Routine (FAR) occurs when you go into your patient's room to do your first full head-to-toe assessment of the day. Here's what I like to do for my FAR:

- Check vital signs
- Perform head-to-toe assessment
- Verify presence of safety equipment (suction tubing, oxygen, and ambu-bag)
- Empty Foley bag
- Untangle and label IV lines; trace line from bag, to pump to patient
- Give the room a quick clean-up
- Check to see which supplies are already in the room
- Reposition patient if needed
- Discuss plan for the day with patient/family

You will also want to have a quick little routine that you perform before you leave the patient's room. I call this a Spot Check as you are just checking for a few simple things:

- Bed low and locked
- Call light within reach
- Bedside table within reach (when appropriate, a sedated patient won't be using a bedside table, but an alert patient will)
- Urinal within reach
- Before leaving the room, I ask the patient what I can bring

the next time I come in the room and let them know when I will return. "I'll be back in about 30 minutes, is there anything you need right now?" This really reduces call lights if the patient knows you're coming back and you will bring their coffee, extra blanket, newspaper, etc... If they have an urgent need (pain is a big one), of course you'll take care of that right away.

And, of course, you will have an End-of-Shift Routine but that doesn't mean it has to occur right at the end of the day. Saving things until the last minute is usually a guarantee you'll get out late. I start my EOS at around 1700 (report starts at 1845) and it consists of the following:

- Calculate intake & output
- Look through the day's orders one more time, make a list of things I must pass off to the next shift
- Ensure IV bags won't run out at change-of-shift; if anything is close to empty, change it out now or at least get a replacement bag ready to go (there's nothing more annoying than starting your shift with empty bags, so be nice to the nurse following you)
- Give the room a quick clean-up if I haven't done so already
- Reposition patient one last time
- Catch up on charting vital signs
- Make sure paperwork is all in order and where it's supposed to be
- Prepare to give report

The Daily Flow

As far as developing routines go, my workday typically flows the same each day, but "situations" will always throw a kink into things. I would say the morning is much more predictable usually, and as the day progresses it's a little more loosey-goosey. In general, let's assume you've got Patient A who is super sick, on a vent and has titratable gtts ("gtt" is nursey talk for "drip" meaning you've got an IV infusion of something important like insulin, levophed or cardizem), and Patient B who isn't so bad off and will probably transfer out in the next day or so. The day pretty much looks like this:

0645-0715: Get report, greet both patients/families, super quick focused assessment (if they're in for neuro, do a quick neuro check...if they're in for respiratory, then check O2 sat, respiratory effort, ask about shortness of breath...if they're post surgical, ask about pain, see if there are pools of blood in the bed, look at the dressing, you get the idea). Ask each patient what I can bring them when I come back for their assessment. By asking what you can bring the patient THE NEXT TIME you come in, I find it cuts down on the waitressing aspect of the job.

0715-0730: SOS Routine. Fill pockets (end-caps and alcohol swabs, make sure I have at least three pens, a hemostat, scissors and my steth); Print EKG strips, take a quick look at labs, check to see if I need to replace K or Mg, write out my schedule of meds, lab draws, TODO items; Grab the warm blanket Patient B asked for earlier; He's on sliding scale insulin and looks hungry, so I'll get the glucometer and his tray unless my other patient needs me RIGHT NOW. Otherwise, I can take 3 minutes for a quick accu-check and meal delivery.

0730-0800: First Assessment Routine (FAR). Assess sick Patient A first and TRY to chart it on the flowsheet. If she's a typical ICU patient, then she has CVP and possibly A-Lines to level, waveforms to print, gtts to titrate, may need a turn and oral care if on vent...again, cluster cluster cluster (remember your High Fives!) While I'm in the room for this first assessment, I'll do a quick survey of what supplies are already in there, what supplies I need to bring THE NEXT TIME I go in. I'll also update patient/family on the general plan and goals for the day, also find out if there is anything super important to them (maybe they want to nap later because they were up all night, or maybe they want to go outside to the patio, maybe their goal is to ambulate to the toilet for a proper BM...whatever it is, find out and see how you can work it into the day).

One more thing I try to do early is to label all my IV lines and pumps. We have pumps that scroll the name of the drug across the display. Usually I do not have time to wait the four seconds it takes for the name of the drug to scroll across, so I label the pumps, too. Having your IV lines labeled is SUPER IMPORTANT! Trace each bag to its pump then to the patient. Make sure everything is what it's supposed to be, and that nothing incompatible is running together. CLEARLY label each line directly above the Y-site. If there's a "situation," you want to know ASAP which line can be used to push epinephrine, for instance (and it's not your insulin gtt line, so make labeling a part of your daily routine!) Once I've completed my assessment, I'll start making a "problem list." If they're doing pretty good and don't have a lot of problems, then I'll just start a list of things to bring up during rounds.

0800-0830: First Assessment Routine for Patient B. If your patients aren't too terribly ill, this may go a bit quicker, but I try not to stress if it takes me until 0830 to fully assess and chart the assessment on both patients. Remember, I've peeked in at Patient B already and would know if he were in distress, but he's sitting in the bedside chair watching the news, so he's good. Depending on what meds he has, I may be able to administer his 0900 meds now thanks to the hour window available for med passes.

0830-0930: If Patient A has URGENT needs that the doc needs to address, I'll call him as soon as I have all the data I need (lab values, etc.) Otherwise, it's time for morning meds for Patient A, then meds for Patient B if I didn't sneak them in already. As far as meds go, you have to use your judgment. Let's say Patient A is in for septic shock and has scheduled antibiotics at 0900, that's obviously going to take precedence over Patient B's daily Pepcid tablet. Also, you'll want to be sure to look at what antibiotics you have that are all due AT THE SAME TIME. It's amazing how often this happens, and if you have the "Big Daddy" ones that hang for 60-120 minutes, this can be problematic. Sometimes you'll have to check IV compatibility and see what you can flow in together so you can get those antibiotics in ON TIME, ya'll! If I have a patient on a ton of IV meds and I notice when making my schedule that it's going to be tricky to time them out, I will print out an "IV compatibility" report to see ahead of time what I can run together. I put a copy by the bedside and a copy with my paperwork. Super helpful!

0930-1000: Get ready for rounds! We have a list of items that we address in the same format each time, so I just go through the list and write out my notes. This takes a few minutes prep, but makes rounds go super fast. This is also where my problem list comes in handy. If my patient is in dire need of something, I obviously won't wait until rounds to bring it up to the doc. But for less urgent things, I can get a handful of issues all handled at once while the team is rounding. If I have time here, I'll write my narrative notes if I didn't do it earlier when I charted on the flowsheet. If I haven't peaked at my patient's H&P yet I will do it here...sometimes you find tidbits that got missed in report. MAYBE, just maybe I'll go reheat my morning coffee.

1000-1400: Rounds (anywhere from 1000-1200), maybe a morning break and at this point I'm basically on my schedule, doing things like repositioning my patient, providing oral care, giving meds, drawing labs. If I have to travel with my patient (go to CT scan or MRI), I try to get that out of the way ASAP because it will seriously throw a kink into the day. I also try to take lunch by 1400...it is usually possible :-)

1400-1700: By now the docs have rounded and you have orders. If I had STAT orders that I saw earlier, I hopefully have done them by now. Otherwise, it takes a bit for the orders to get processed, but I usually have my charts back by now and can make sure everything has been entered correctly, see what I need to add to my TODO list, and see what will have to be passed along to my friends on the next shift. This is also the time when I do all my "extra fun paperwork" such as care plans, teaching checklist and such. If I have time, I take a more detailed look at my patient's chart so I can see if anything else got missed in report such as test results, past medical stuff, whatever.

1700-1845: EOS Routine. This is when I do my intake & output totals, clear my pumps, empty Foley bag, empty drains, give my room a last minute cleaning, write my end-of-shift summaries, check any pending labs that need to be communicated in report and basically just start buttoning things up.

1845: It's MAGIC TIME! Give report, clock out, go home, RELAX!

Of course, this is an example of a predictable day with patients who are basically cruising along. You can pretty much count on things kinking up your plan, whether it's a transfer out, an admit from the ED, hemodynamic instability, a code, whatever. In general this is how I try to organize my schedule, hopefully leaving enough room to account for the unexpected happening…because it will!

Prioritizing

As students, it is super easy for you to focus on tasks and not see "the big picture." And no worries, that's exactly what's expected of you. But, in order to make the successful transition into new graduate RN you'll need to start thinking more globally, and the sooner the better. Here are some tips.

I always advocate students come up with a schedule for the day. My daily schedules as a student were insane, seriously down to five-minute blocks. As I gained more experience, my schedules became looser and by the time I started working as an RN the schedule listed what I needed to do each hour. These days I go off more of a "to-do" list, but those early days of actually scheduling out my time were invaluable. With that said, a schedule doesn't mean you can throw prioritizing out the window. While a schedule will help you with your time management, prioritizing is a dynamic activity that takes place continually throughout your day. And yes, many times, prioritizing means re-thinking your schedule as you go, making adjustments and acting accordingly. Things to consider as you prioritize throughout your day:

- Who is your most critical patient?
- How long will a specific task take?
- What is the most important piece of data you need now?
- Are you prepared for the unexpected?
- What are your patient's needs, what will serve them best?

Who is your most critical patient?

The thing about this question, is that it can change throughout the day. Just because patient A starts off as your sickest patient, doesn't mean things will stay that way. Maybe patient A will stabilize and patient B will start showing signs of respiratory failure. Now, who's your most critical patient? Understanding that you may need to adjust your focus based on changes in patient condition is imperative to being a good nurse.

How long will a specific task take?

Considering how long a task will take vs. other things you need to do will help you keep the most amount of time available for the most important tasks. Let's say your patient is sitting in the chair and wants to get back to bed. You know it's going to be a group project and will likely take a while. In the meantime, your other patient is on an insulin gtt and needs a blood sugar taken every hour otherwise they might get more insulin than they need, which would be extremely dangerous. It is OK to tell your chair patient, "I need to go take care of one quick thing, then I'll bring someone to help me get you back to bed." Not getting bogged down in time-consuming tasks when essential things MUST get done is a key to effective prioritizing.

What is the most important piece of data you need right now?

This will vary depending on what is going on with your patient. Let's say you have a fresh craniotomy patient and a patient on a vent. Your orders indicate you are to do hourly neuro checks on your crani patient, and your patient on the vent needs a daily blood gas. Considering that neuro changes can occur very quickly, you'd want to conduct your neuro check first. The blood gas, though important, is a daily task and can probably wait the five minutes you need to conduct a neuro assessment on your more critical patient. If your patient is on vasoactive medication to raise or lower their blood pressure, you want to know their blood pressure at all times. If he's in renal failure, you'll be eying his urine output like a hawk. Knowing what key data you need at any given time will help you prioritize what needs to be done/assessed in relation to everything else you have going on.

Are you prepared for the unexpected?

Knowing what potential crisis could occur, can make you keen to what your priorities for the day are and help you be prepared. For example, knowing that your patient presented to the ED in complete heart block and that your other patient is at huge risk for cerebral vasospasm put you in the mind-set of being ready for (and assessing appropriately for) any disasters coming your way. I always start my shift with a little "what if," and a plan for what I can do to prevent it and react to it.

What are your patient's needs and what will serve them best?

Each patient will need different things based on their pathophysiological process. Knowing what these needs and priorities are will help you keep the most important things at the forefront. For example, let's say you have a septic patient whose K is 3.3, Mg is 1.8 and has multiple IV meds due at 0900...vanco, potassium, magnesium and a banana bag. You've only got one available IV site (your other two sites are being hogged by an insulin gtt and bicarb gtt)...what meds are you going to give first? Remember he's septic, so you're going to give the antibiotics first every single time. If his K were 2.6 and he were having cardiac problems, you'd need to either give it PO or start another line because sometimes prioritizing means doing two things at once. I've always said I'd be Super Nurse if only I had three hands and ten IV lines.

A Word About Safety

Being safe is the absolute most important priority of any nursing student (or nurse). I have seen students attempt to perform tasks on their own, thinking it will make them seem confident and self-sufficient (this usually ends badly). I have seen students completely oblivious to high-priority alarms (how anyone could tune out that awful racket is beyond me), and I have witnessed students taking FOREVER to reattach a pulse oximetry probe to a patient in respiratory failure. I about crawled out of my skin on that one.

I once had a student who was attempting to reposition an intubated and restrained patient without letting me know or even getting help from the patient mobility tech (lift team). I was alerted to this fiasco by the sound of the ventilator alarm and the oxygen saturation alarm going off at the same time. Luckily, I was right outside the room. When I entered, I spotted my student just staring at the monitor as it dinged and clanged, patient flat, tube feed still running, and the student just standing there frozen. Why the student didn't immediately call out for help, I have no idea. Trying to save face? Maybe. Not sure what to do? Probably. The point is, the patient could have suffered immensely. His oxygen levels were down, he was at huge risk for aspiration because the tube feed was not placed on hold during the position change, the patient was restrained and was at high risk for self-extubation. The list goes on and on as to why this student should have never tried to take on this task without an RN there to supervise. Even seasoned nurses will not reposition a vented patient without someone else there to watch the ventilator tubing and IV lines. As the preceptor, it is my job to keep both the patient and the student safe. I immediately stopped the tube feeding as I returned the patient to an upright position, gave him extra oxygen and stayed at the bedside until things stabilized. I then spoke to my student, explaining why this should never ever in a hundred-million-years ever happen again. The moral of the story? Ask for help, ask for guidance. Use your head and try to anticipate all the things that could go wrong so you can recognize high-risk situations that require an extra set of more-experienced hands.

In addition to the things your school requires you to do only with supervision, I recommend always asking your RN to accompany you when performing the following:

> • Suctioning an intubated patient
> • Suctioning a patient with a tracheostomy, ESPECIALLY a new one. Actually, do not even touch a fresh tracheostomy, don't even look at it (ok, just kidding, you can look at it). Fresh tracheostomies are at high risk for becoming dislodged, and if this happens it is a very bad day for everyone involved.
> • Hanging any IV medication
> • Adjusting the drip rate of any potent medication such as vasoactive meds, insulin, beta blockers, etc...
> • Repositioning any patient with the following: vent, chest tube, multiple drains, large surgical wounds, back surgeries, cervical injuries, hemodynamic instability, respiratory issues
> • Never silence another nurse's monitor alarm. EVER.

Communicating in Clinical using SBAR

SBAR is a standardized method of communicating quickly and efficiently to other members of the healthcare team.

> *S: Situation* - Why are you calling? What is going on with your patient that has you so concerned you are calling a neurologist

in the middle of the night or interrupting your RN during her break?

B: Background - A brief background that is relevant to your patient's condition at this time.

A: Assessment - Vital signs, physical assessment findings, lab results, whatever it is that you've assessed about the patient that is your cause for concern or may be relevant to the situation.

R: Recommendation - Your recommendation to the physician (or your RN). This is where you ask for specific orders or discuss what you think the patient needs. As students, you will not be allowed to take phone orders, but you can still use SBAR to convey your concerns to the RN you're working with for the day. In some cases your RN may allow you to use SBAR with a physician provided s/he is there with you and the physician is willing to write the order (and not insist you take a verbal order).

We'll do an easy one first. Let's say your patient is complaining of nausea, but has nothing ordered medication wise. The MD is on the unit so you and the RN approach her with your SBAR communication ready to go:

S: Situation - Hi, Dr. Saylors, I'm a nursing student working with Alexis. I have a request for Carolina Freeman.

B: Background - She had a total abdominal hysterectomy yesterday,

A: Assessment - and is complaining of severe nausea; she has not been able to tolerate her clear liquid diet.

R: Recommendation - Could we get an order for an anti-emetic please?

You see how straight, quick and to-the-point it is? No need to go off on a big rambling story as doctor's minds just don't tend to work that way. Add to that the fact that physicians get interrupted and called all day and all night, and you'll understand the need to be brief. Believe me, if the MD wants more information, she'll ask specific questions. Here's another one: Your patient is experiencing hypotension after her surgery and your RN is at break. You go to the charge nurse with your SBAR report.

S: Situation - Excuse me, Charlene. I need to talk with you about Cheri Davis, a 66-year-old patient of Dr. Wilson's. I'm concerned about her blood pressure.

B: Background - She had a colectomy this morning and has a baseline blood pressure in the 120s, an echo done two weeks ago shows an ejection fraction of 65%.

A: Assessment - Her BP is currently 82/43, HR 114, RR 24 and O2 sat 90% on 4L NC. She's complaining of feeling short-of-breath and slightly dizzy.

R: Recommendation - Can you come see this patient? I think we should notify the MD to see about a fluid bolus and a CBC. She may also benefit from transfer to the ICU.

In this scenario, you're worried about your patient's blood pressure. You are letting the charge nurse know right away that the patient had surgery just that day, and that her baseline blood pressure and cardiac function were normal. You then go on to tell her "just the facts" and then make a recommendation. In some cases, your recommendation will be spot-on, other times it will be way off base. You'll get better at it, it just takes time and experience. The person you are reporting to (nurse, respiratory therapist, MD) may also quiz you about other factors before moving forward. For instance, if you hadn't told the nurse about the patient's ejection fraction, she may have inquired about the patient's history in this regard because you don't want to be giving a patient with congestive heart failure a big ol' fluid bolus. As you gain experience, you'll anticipate the questions that are likely to be asked and gather data accordingly.

One more easy one. Your patient is a 52-year-old truck driver with a history of asthma. On your morning head-to-toe assessment you notice audible expiratory wheezes in the upper airways and he states his chest feels "tight." You see the respiratory therapist strolling by with her mug of coffee and you get your SBAR ready:

S: Situation - Good morning Stephanie, I'm worried about Mr. Richards in 5324.

B: Background - He came in through the ED yesterday for fever, they're working him up for pneumonia. He has a history of asthma and he smokes a pack a day.

A: Assessment - He has expiratory wheezes in the upper lobes and is complaining of a tight feeling in his chest.

R: Recommendation - Can you come listen to him and see if it's appropriate for him to have his prn albuterol now?

OK, now that we've done a few "easy" ones, let's try one that's a little more involved. Your patient has a diagnosis of ischemic stroke. He came in through the ED that afternoon complaining of left-sided weakness and slurred speech. After a CT scan confirmed he was not bleeding into his brain, he was given a clot-busting drug and shuttled off to the ICU for close monitoring and hourly neuro exams. As you are conducting your 1500 assessment, you notice your previously alert and oriented patient is no longer following commands. He is withdrawing to pain on upper extremities only and his left pupil is larger than his right. You notice a gurgling in his airway because he is unable to cough effectively. Your communication to the RN might go something like this:

> *S: Situation* - Excuse me, Anthony. I'm concerned about Ricardo Juarez in room 5203. He's had a change in neuro status.
>
> *B: Background* - He's the patient that received TPA this morning for ischemic stroke and experienced resolution of his neuro symptoms until just now when changes were noted.
>
> *A: Assessment* - His left pupil is larger than the right and he is no longer following commands; withdrawal to pain on upper extremities only. He has no cough and secretions are audible in oropharynx. O2 sats are down to 88% on 4L NC, respiratory therapy is at the bedside now.
>
> *R: Recommendation* - I think he needs to be intubated for airway protection, and he should probably go for a STAT CT scan and we should draw coags, too. Can we go see him and ask the doc to come to the bedside now?

In this scenario, the physician and RN need to come to the bedside now to assess this awful deterioration in neuro status. Notice how we use the phrase "I'm concerned" in this example and "I'm worried" in the previous one. Both phrases convey a sense of urgency when it is needed. No need to use those words for routine orders for pain medicine and such, but when the physician or RN needs to intervene right away, you darn well better paint a picture of just how dire the situation is.

Be Organized and Tidy

One of the very first things I teach my students is that I consider organization and tidiness to be just as important as skills mastery. That's because an organized and tidy work area is a safe work area, and I am all about patient safety (and I know you are, too).

To illustrate my point, picture a room with clutter on every available surface, IV lines an unlabeled and tangled mess, paperwork in a chaotic stack, extra linens stacked hither and yon, a full sharps container, alcohol swabs and various other litter scattered across the floor, last night's dinner tray emitting the odor of food cooked 17 hours ago, filthy suction tubing coated with secretions, and overflowing garbage bins stuffed with foul-smelling waste. If you think I am exaggerating, I can assure you I am not. I have seen it more times than I care to count, and there are two reasons a room like this is absolutely not okay.

For starters, no patient deserves to live in filth and chaos. These people are sick, they are recuperating, they are stressed, they are often depressed and they have very little control over their lives at this time. Do you really think they want to live like this, even if for just a few days? Secondly, does this room seem safe to you? What if there were an emergent situation? Do you even have room to work? Do you know which IV lines are available if you need to give emergency medication? What are you going to do with your sharps since the container is full? Do you have instant and immediate access to the data needed to handle the situation, or did you leave your paperwork laying around in some random spot or in a haphazard pile at your workstation? Leaving your workspace an absolute disaster conveys a message, and probably not the one you want to convey. It says that you don't take pride in your work, don't care about the comfort or dignity of your patient and basically that you're lazy. Granted, there are busy shifts where the shilolah does hit the fan...but that should be the exception and not the rule.

Now picture a room clear of clutter, supplies organized and placed in cabinets, IV lines labeled, paperwork in order, garbage bins and sharps containers available for use, the air smells clean and your patient is tidy. Which room would you rather work in? Which room do you think your patient would rather live in? As a student, this is the perfect time for you to begin practicing good habits. But you may be wondering how on earth you are going to fit all this tidying-up and organizing into your already busy day. I always try to do a little first thing in the morning, before things get intense. At the very least I'll label my lines when I'm doing my initial assessment (since verifying lines is part of your assessment.) Then, throughout the morning I'll do a little each time I go in, and if I have time to commit 15 minutes to it, I'll just take care of it all at once. After that, it's easy to keep your room clean. You just CYAG (clean as you go) and voila...the end of your shift arrives and your patient and room are as fresh and tidy as a new admission! Next thing you know, your stress levels drop, your workflow is greatly improved, you can find what you need when you need it, and nurses look forward to following you from shift to shift :-)

CHAPTER EIGHT

STUDY GROUPS

Now this is where I am really going to blow your mind. Study groups are a waste of time. A monumental waste of time. Getting together with four, five, or even six other students is a surefire way to get very little accomplished and necessitate missing out on sleep in order to get caught up. There are two reasons study groups just don't work. The first reason is that the chances of finding five or six people who all study the exact same way is practically nil. The second reason, is that they quickly run the risk of turning into social hour, gripe sessions and gossip circles. You do not have time for this.

Notice I'm not saying you should avoid studying with others. If you find one or two other people you gel with, then I do think it can be beneficial to get together to quiz each other or work on projects. If your school uses online quizzes, and your instructor has given advance approval to do the quizzes as a group, doing them with a max of three people can be very helpful. I'd actually recommend just working in pairs, but some people just can't get away from the "study group" mentality. By working in pairs, you get the opportunity to see more of the question bank and discuss together the rationales for all the correct and incorrect answers. You can also jam through your quizzes pretty quickly.

Not yet convinced? Picture seven people getting together to do an online quiz consisting of 10 questions. If each question takes a total of three minutes to read, research, ponder and answer, that means each quiz is going to take thirty minutes. Let's assume each person in the group gets a new bank of questions (not likely, but for argument's sake) and now we're looking at three-and-a-half hours to essentially get ONE item crossed off your Master Schedule. Even if the test bank questions were limited and some questions were repeated, maybe your subsequent quiz takers would average two minutes per question. It would still take you two-and-a-half hours to take one quiz. Factor in that you will have many weeks where you could potentially have seven or more quizzes to take (on top of everything else), and now you're looking at a total of more than 17 hours a week just on quizzes. And that's without your group doing any socializing at all. You do not have time for this. Believe me now?

If you are going to study with others, I recommend working in pairs or three people at the absolute most. Have a clear plan for what you are going to study and how you are going to do it. Are you going to discuss case studies, quiz each other on fundamentals, go over NCLEX questions or take turns teaching each other a subject that's going to be on the exam? By having a clear idea of the goals of the group, you'll actually get some studying done and maximize your time effectively. Anything else is an unfortunate and regrettable waste of time.

CHAPTER NINE

TEST-TAKING STRATEGIES

Nursing school exams are weird. There, I said it. You will, however, get used to the weirdness if you know what to expect and try not to let it frustrate you too much. The reason nursing school exams are so odd is because the instructors need to get you used to a very particular type of question that will help you develop critical thinking skills and prepare for your licensing exam (NCLEX).

NCLEX-Style Questions

The maddening thing about NCLEX-style questions, is that they will often have four correct answers, but one MOST correct answer. See how frustrating that can be? It's not like typical multiple-choice questions where you can just find the right answer and move on. With NCLEX-style questions you must think through the rationale for each answer and see which one is most correct. The answers also require critical thinking skills where you use applied knowledge, and not just regurgitate the right answer.

For example, a question isn't going to say, "What are the classic signs of delirium?" Instead, the question will want you to use your knowledge of delirium in order to answer appropriately. If this doesn't make sense right now, don't worry…you'll see what I mean soon enough. Here are a few things to keep in mind as you answer these questions.

- Life or death situations
- Patient safety
- Focus on teaching/learning
- The nursing process
- What issues need to be addressed first (prioritizing)
- Acute vs. chronic
- The patient's developmental stage

Life or Death Situations (think of your ABCs).

Q: Your stroke patient is suddenly unresponsive, he will not follow commands and his breathing is labored. You want to:

A) do a thorough neuro exam
B) send him to CT scan STAT
C) intubate him and place on a ventilator
D) draw a stat CBC, PTT and INR (coagulation studies)

In this case, you would do ALL of those things, but there is one thing you would do before any of the others and that is intubate your patient. An unresponsive patient is at huge risk for respiratory failure. Airway wins, and it's the A in your ABC (airway, breathing, circulation).

Patient Safety

Q: Your patient is complaining of pain 9/10 in abdomen, breathing 36 times a minute and writhing in bed. She is moaning and agitated, pulling at her gown. HR is 124, BP is 163/112, O2 saturation is 91% on RA. You decide to:

A) Place an oxygen mask on the patient, instruct her to take calm deep breaths.
B) Administer two pain pills with plenty of water
C) Administer medication to lower her blood pressure
D) Call the MD and ask for an order for IV pain medication

The correct answer is D. You do not want to give a patient who is breathing that fast anything to swallow as the risk for aspiration is high. Though you do want to provide oxygen for this patient, she is not likely to tolerate a mask as she is already pulling at her gown. You would not give blood pressure medication at this time, as controlling her pain is more important...once the pain is controlled, the blood pressure is likely to come down as well. See how all the answers are correct (or close to correct), but one is MORE correct? That's how the NCLEX works.

Focus on Teaching/Learning

Q: Your patient is a 25-year-old female who presented to the ED six hours ago with a blood sugar of 695. She is diagnosed as a Type 1 diabetic and placed on an insulin infusion and transferred to the ICU. She cries when you check her blood sugar saying, "I don't want to have diabetes." To help her learn about her diagnosis you:

A) Ask her what she knows about diabetes
B) Calmly explain how to use the glucometer to check her blood sugar and ask her for a return demonstration
C) Print out information on diabetes management and leave it at her bedside
D) Request that a member of the hospital's diabetes support group visit the patient

Many questions will focus on evaluating your patient for their education needs. The correct answer is A. Prior to doing any teaching, you must ascertain what your patient knows so you can tailor your teaching specifically. While you would want to show her how to use the glucometer, this is not the time to do it as she would not be receptive to teaching at this time of high anxiety. Printing out information on diabetes is a good idea, but you wouldn't want to just leave it on the bedside table. The patient will need extensive teaching that cannot be accomplished passively. Answer D is also a good idea, but this can occur later when the patient is more receptive.

The Nursing Process

Q: Your patient is a 57-year-old man with a history of smoking, pneumonia and COPD. He tells you he's feeling anxious about his breathing, so you...

A) Administer an anti-anxiety medication
B) Assess his O2 saturation level
C) Put him on a high-flow oxygen mask
D) Teach him a pursed-lip breathing technique

Some questions will want you to use the nursing process to know what you're going to do for your patient. The first step in the nursing process is assessment, so answer B is the correct answer. While most of the other answers are correct, answer B is the MOST correct. Just FYI, you wouldn't want to put a patient with COPD on a high-flow oxygen mask as too much oxygen can knock out their respiratory drive. With COPD patients, you use the least amount of oxygen needed to achieve an O2 level of around 88-90%. Answer D is not the desired action at this time, since trying to teach someone while they're anxious is futile.

What issues need to be addressed first?

> Q: You receive report at 0645 on four patients. Your assignment for the day includes a 45-year old woman who had a below-the-knee amputation yesterday and is complaining of 6/10 pain, a 85 year-old blind man with dementia and left-sided weakness who is climbing out of bed, a 32-year old man with cellulitis of the leg who needs to be prepped for a 10:00 surgery, and a 53-year old woman recovering from back surgery who needs help ambulating to the toilet. Who do you attend to first?

> A) Medicate your amputation patient for pain while you have the nurse's aid help the back surgery patient get to the toilet
> B) Help the 85-year old dementia patient use the urinal then get him back to bed
> C) Greet your cellulitis patient and begin the pre-surgical prep list, delegate the dementia patient to your nurse's aid
> D) Ask the nurse's aid to help the dementia patient while you ambulate the back surgery patient to the toilet

Some questions will ask you which patient you are going to see first. As you get more adept at prioritizing, these questions will get more complex. In this case, you are going to choose answer B as it is the only answer that addresses the most urgent need first. In this case, the most urgent need is patient safety. At first glance, answer C looks promising, since it addresses the need for patient safety through the delegation of tasks. What answer C does not address is the next most urgent need, and that's your patient in 6/10 pain. Besides, notice that it's only 7:00 and surgery isn't coming for your patient until 10:00, you've got time to do the checklist a little later. In a perfect world, you would medicate the patient who's in pain while the nurse's aid helps the dementia patient, but that would have been too easy.

Acute vs Chronic

Q: Your 87-year old patient with a 30-year history of COPD is complaining of a headache 7/10. Her oxygen saturation level is 89% on 2L nasal cannula. She is alert, oriented and able to speak in full sentences. You listen to your patient's lungs and notice diminished breath sounds in all lobes. Your next course of action is to:

A) Increase the oxygen on her nasal cannula
B) Call the doctor for a stat portable chest x-ray
C) Page the respiratory therapist
D) Treat the headache with 1 mg morphine IV

Some questions will want you to think about acute vs chronic problems. In this case, the correct answer is D. The patient's respiratory problems are chronic as evidenced by her history of COPD. Long-term COPD patients are absolutely fine at an oxygen level of 89%, so this is a bit of a trick question. In most cases, the respiratory intervention would supersede almost anything else, but in this case we're going to treat her acute condition, the headache.

The Patient's Developmental Stage

Q: You are taking care of a 16-year old girl with new-onset diabetes. She has been withdrawn the past two days, and seems depressed. When you go in to perform her lunchtime blood sugar test, you notice she has barely moved since your last assessment. As a super nurse you are going to say:

A) "I know someone with diabetes and she is doing just fine."
B) "Why don't you call a few of your friends and have them come by for a visit. We can practice injecting your insulin with your evening dose."
C) "I have a small doll we can practice giving insulin injections to. Would you like that?"
D) "This depression isn't helping matters. I'm going to have the social worker come speak with you."

Many questions will have you take the patient's developmental stage into account. In this case, the answer is B. As you will learn in your pediatrics course, social networks are one of the most important things to a teenager. Having her friends by for a visit could do wonders for her mood and outlook.

Answer A does not acknowledge the patient's feelings, answer C would be more appropriate for a small child and answer D absolves the nurse from all responsibility and puts the blame on the patient. But at first glance they all seem like really awesome things to say, don't they? That's how the NCLEX questions get you...they trick you into saying, "I'd do ALL those things" or in some cases, "I wouldn't do ANY of that!" You just have to find the answer that's more correct than all the others. You'll love it.

In general, the best way to prepare for NCLEX-style exams is to get yourself an NCLEX prep book. It may seem strange to start studying for your licensing exam as a first semester nursing student, but these books are excellent tools to help you study for your exams. Look for a book that has questions organized by body system, and make sure you find one that lists the rationales for all answers (the correct ones as well as the incorrect ones.)

Your Test Day Game Plan

If you've been studying the *Straight A* way, you are absolutely, positively ready for your exam. You have been quizzing yourself using flashcards, NCLEX books and audio files, plus you got a good night's rest the night before. It is now test day and you want to do your absolute best. Heed this advice and you will. I promise.

The first strategy for test day success is to avoid studying on test day. This was mentioned before, but it bears repeating because the temptation to study on exam day is going to be huge. Everyone else will be cramming at the last minute, quizzing each other, freaking out and generally causing themselves a lot of stress and chaos. You are going to find a quiet place to relax before your exam, even if it's just around the corner from the exam room...just get away from all the madness. I recommend listening to music, but if other relaxation technique works better for you, by all means go for it: meditation, calling your uncle, looking at pictures of your dog, going for a walk or perhaps doing a crossword puzzle. Just do something to clear your mind and make you feel peaceful so you can walk into your test the confident, rockstar nurse that you are.

Most exams in nursing school are computer based. Again, this is to prep you for your ultimate computer-based exam, the NCLEX. When you sit down at the computer, take a quick moment to make sure the keyboard and mouse work. There's nothing more anxiety-provoking than fiddling with a computer that doesn't work while all your classmates are busily logging into the test while you flounder away wasting precious time.

Once you're logged in and you know everything works, close your eyes, take three deep breaths and say to yourself, 'I know this material, I know this material, I know this material." Open your eyes and click on the first question. Read the question but don't look at the answer. Try to determine what the question is asking before you go off looking at the answers. Remember, the answers are there to distract you, so you want to be sure you know what the question is asking before you start getting distracting by all the incorrect answers that sound so good. I like to keep a piece of scratch paper next to my computer. For each question, I write out "a, b, c, d" and cross them off one at a time as I eliminate the incorrect answers. As you go through each multiple-choice option, think through the rational for each one…why it's right or why it's wrong. If you are lucky, you will pretty quickly be able to get it down to two options. In some cases you'll feel like you're guessing, but what's really happening is you are using your nursey instinct. It's like spidey-sense but much, much better.

As you go through your exam, there will be questions you simply cannot answer. Prior to starting your exam, the instructor will let you know if the test allows you to go back and change answers or revisit questions. If your exam allows you to do this and you come across a question you don't know the answer to, go ahead and select your best guess and write down the question number so you can come back to it later. Once you are finished with the exam, go back through all the questions you were unsure about. The reason you don't want to dwell too long on any one question as you are initially going through the test is because your tests will be timed. Again, this is to prepare you for your NCLEX. If seeing the time click click click away from you causes more anxiety, check to see if the test allows you to hide the timer. You can always go back and un-hide it if you need to see how much time you have left.

So by now you have gone through the entire test once, gone back to revisit a handful of questions a second time and you've still got twenty minutes left on your exam. My strategy was always to go back through one more time and just reiterate that I answered everything correctly. If you have used your scratch paper, you can even look to make sure you selected the answer you intended to select. The danger with going back through the test one more time is that you might feel inclined to change answers. Usually, if you're unsure about an answer, it's best to go with your initial instinct. However, there are times when a question further on in the test provides you with information that can be utilized to answer a question elsewhere in the exam. If this occurs, and it's a major revelation that changes your answer, by all means change it, but only if you're sure.

Once you are finished with your exam, leave the testing room and go on about your day. The temptation to stick around and wait for your classmates so you can compare answers will be great, but it will only cause you more anxiety. Depending on what else you have going on that day, this might be a wonderful time to take a short break to do something enjoyable. I'm not talking about taking the whole afternoon off, but maybe you could meet a friend for coffee, take your dog out for a run, or watch an episode of Grey's Anatomy and criticize all the medical inaccuracies (like doctor's spending all their time at the bedside and hanging IV fluids).

Skills Check Off
Your lab classes will require that you get checked off on certain skills. They will range from the simple such as taking an accurate blood pressure to the more complex such as performing a neurological evaluation or starting an IV. My first skills check-off had me in such a tizzy that I arranged to meet a friend before class so we could go through every single little step in advance. I even wrote out a script so that I wouldn't miss any critical components. Once I got this first skills check-off under my belt, I didn't have to write out scripts but I would still practice ahead of time.

Prior to your skills check-off, your professor will provide you with information regarding the criteria on which you will be graded. Use this as a guide as you practice. For instance, if forgetting to perform hand hygiene is an automatic fail, you'll want to be sure you incorporate this step every single time you practice.

Typically, your check-off will involve you going into the exam area one at a time, just you and the professor. S/he typically won't say anything, you are expected to know what to do and how to do it. Take your time, pay close attention to critical elements such as performing hand hygiene, keeping a sterile field and putting on gloves. Your instructor is looking to see if you are able to safely perform the skill on an actual patient, meaning you will keep them from harm by following all procedures carefully. Most schools will give you two chances to pass a skills check-off, so try not to fret too much if you don't pass your first time. Learn from your mistakes and move on.

Some of your skills check-offs will take place in clinical. For example, your professor may want to observe you passing PO meds before letting you loose to perform this skill unsupervised. I remember the first time I performed a blood glucose check on a patient under the watchful eye of my scary-as-heck nursing professor. I got all the way to the part where I was about to prick my patient's finger with the lancet when my professor reminded me I had not put on gloves. So, sometimes you'll forget to do the most basic thing. Believe me, I never forgot to put gloves on after that, and passed my second attempt with flying colors. No worries, you'll do great.

CHAPTER TEN

GROUP PROJECTS

Nursing professors love group projects. They absolutely love them. Students, on the other hand, absolutely hate them. So I guess it all evens out.

You will do an inordinate number of group projects in nursing school, possibly four or more each semester. The problem with group projects is that the weight of the tasks is never evenly divided, and it's the group leader who usually gets the short end of the stick. To divide the work equitably, you must first understand the key roles in any group project. The good news is there are basically just two: group leader and worker bee.

> • Group Leader: Organizes the project timeline, harasses people for their assignments, puts the entire project together (such as a Power Point presentation or APA-formatted paper), acts as a resource person and problem-solver for the entire project, and edits the entire paper so it all uses consistent and error-free language.

> • Worker Bees: Each bee takes a segment of the project.

Easy enough, right? The key to being a good worker bee is getting your assignment to the group leader on time and in the format agreed upon by the group. Make sure you include your references (in proper format) so that all the leader has to do is cut and paste them together.

To make your group project run smoothly, do the following as soon as your group is formed:

• Appoint a group leader. This is best if it's the person with excellent organizational skills, solid writing ability and has an eye for making things look professional. As the group leader, do not be tempted to take on a portion of the project. It may seem like your task is the easiest, but I guarantee you will be putting in twice as much time as anyone else. If someone fails to do their portion, it falls upon the group leader to pick up the slack. Sad but true.

• Define the tasks of the project. This can range from researching and writing a section, performing interviews, spearheading community outreach, etc... Whatever it may be, just do your best to divide the tasks evenly. Nothing grows group animosity more than members who get off easy and just sit back and watch as their classmates scramble to get things done.

• Define the format in which everyone will submit their work. If it's a paper, you may require everyone submit it as a Word document in Times New Roman, with references properly listed. If it's a PowerPoint presentation, have everyone use a plain white background with black text in the same font so that it's easy for the group leader to add color and graphics. This is not time to get fancy as the leader will just have to reformat everything. Keep it simple.

• Develop a timeline for the project. The group leader will be responsible for putting the whole piece together, and some projects require things be done in a sequential manner so it is imperative that everyone stick to the deadlines. If you're the group leader, feel free to harass people when they are late. As the boss, this is your right and your duty.

• Share contact information. Make sure all members of the group are reachable via phone or email in order to make the sharing of information easy for everyone.

As long as everyone in your group has a clear idea of their role, their due dates and communicates openly with timeliness and respect, your project will go off without a hitch.

CHAPTER ELEVEN

MAKE TIME FOR YOURSELF

Now that you've got the tools you need to be a kick-a$% nursing student, you've got a few extra minutes to spend a little time on yourself. It can be overwhelmingly easy for some of you to devote all your time and attention to school (especially those Type-A personalities), but you will fare better overall if you try to maintain some balance in your life. If you're a planner like me, then schedule these self-care activities into your week. As you may have guessed, I absolutely swear by the audio-quiz technique. Once I started using this tool, I felt absolutely liberated! I could study and still get my chores, laundry, errands and exercise done, which freed me up for a little "me time" once in a while.

Social

Please try to stay in touch with your friends and family. Though you may not see them as often as you did before the madness began, at least shoot for some face-to-face time every couple of weeks or so. Even if it's just to grab a quick cup of coffee in between study sessions, it's important to talk to someone (ANYONE) about something other than nursing school. I remember one year (third semester, maybe) where I actually stopped studying the evening before a test and went to a party. Now, I would never have done this if I wasn't fully prepared, but I could have also stayed home and kept right on studying. Really glad I got out of the house that day...the party was definitely worth it!

Exercise

Please try to stay on top of your exercise. It is an excellent stress reliever and so good for your spirit to do something physical. Nursing school is a very mental activity, so it's good to balance things out with something involving your body, sweat, and preferably the great outdoors. Invite a friend along for a walk or a run, and bam...you've just combined social and exercise into one! Way to multi-task!

Eat Well

Please take care of your body and your brain by eating good food. Nursing school is a very busy time and the temptation to just "grab something" is enormous. If you followed the tips I outlined in the first pages of this book, then hopefully you've got a system in place for eating good, nutritious food even when you're on the run. When I think of the notion of eating well while in school, I remember one night when I had wine and donuts for dinner. Probably not the best choice.

Sleep

Please get the rest you need to function properly. My entire motivation for using good time management and organization skills in school was due to my need for quality sleep each night. That's actually what made me realize rather quickly that study groups were a waste of time. I figured if I spent two hours doing a quiz with my study group when I could finish it in thirty minutes on my own, that I just bought myself an hour-and-a-half of sleep. Sold.

My goal throughout all of school was to be in bed by 11pm. You will come across many a classmate who regularly stays up studying until 2, 3, even 4 in the morning. This does not have to be your reality, especially if you use my tips. Probably the toughest nights to make it to bed on time were clinical prep nights, as those could often take six or seven hours to complete. If I didn't get to the hospital early that day, it was a mad dash to my 11pm deadline, but I managed it and so can you.

THAT'S ALL FOLKS

By the time you are reading this, you are vastly ahead of the curve and well-positioned to do your absolute best in nursing school while holding on to your sanity and your social life.

You are about to embark on one of the most rewarding, demanding and stress-inducing times of your life. I sincerely hope that the tips I have shared with you here will lighten your load considerably, boost your confidence and give you the tools you need to not only survive nursing school, but thrive in nursing school. Please check back in and let me know how you are doing!

Post a comment on the blog - www.straightanursingstudent.com
Chime in on Facebook - www.facebook.com/straightanursingstudent
Shoot me an email - straightanursing@icloud.com

Be safe out there!

-Nurse Mo

p.s. Images, checklists and other resources can be found at the Straight A Nursing Student website at www.straightanursingstudent.com. Enjoy!

APPENDIX A
Commonly Used Abbreviations

Nursing school and the hospital are awash with abbreviations and acronyms. You will spend half your time decoding your patient's chart in the beginning, but soon this shorthand will become second nature. For standard medical acronyms and abbreviations I highly recommend using an app so that you can quickly look them up on the go. There are several such apps out there and most are just 99 cents...well worth it!

In addition, I have compiled a list of commonly-used abbreviations that you might see or wish to use in order to make your note taking a little more efficient. Once on the job (or in clinical), you can use these on your report sheets, but for charting I'd say write things out until you know what's acceptable at your place of work/clinical.

c (with a line over it) = with
s (with a line over it) = without
p (with a line over it) = after
a (with a line over it) before
ac = before meals
pc = after meals
q = every (as in "q day")
hs = hour of sleep, bedtime
prn = as needed
BID = twice a day
TID = three times a day
QID = four times a day
Tx = treatment
Dx = diagnosis
Thx = therapy (pretty sure I made that one up)
Sx = surgery
Rx = pharmacy or prescription
Abx = antibiotics
gtt = drip (as in an IV infusion)
d/t = due to
s/t = secondary to
r/t = related to
s/p = status post (as in "she is s/p appendectomy", she just had surgery)
r/o = rule out

c/o = complains of

s/s = signs & symptoms

a triangle (delta symbol) = change or changes

+/- = with or without, maybe or maybe not, possible

VSS = vital signs stable

WA = while awake

NOC = night shift

APPENDIX B
Resources to Make Your Life Easier

Here are a few resources to make your life as a nursing student easier. Hope they help!

www.bibme.org - This is probably The Best Web Site ever made. It enables you to easily format your references and even save them for future use. Whether it's an online resource, a magazine article, a book or a newspaper story it is super easy to format your sources into the dreaded APA format required by most nursing programs. Be sure to create a profile so you can save them as you will use your references a lot!

https://owl.english.purdue.edu - This is a fantastic resource for writing and includes a whole section on APA format and style.

www.skillstat.com - This website is home to the awesome "6-second ECG" game, in which you try to interpret ECGs as fast as you can (probably the most fun a nursing student could have on a Saturday night). They also publish an e-book on interpreting ECGs...I haven't read it, but anyone who promises a "rapid and reliable" method for interpreting ECGs has my vote. This will come in handy AFTER you've already learned the basics in class.

http://www.aclsmedicaltraining.com/acls-megacode/ - If you are practicing your ACLS, this is a website with a ton of "megacode" scenarios. I didn't take ACLS until after I had graduated, but it's kind of fun to read through the scenarios anyway and get an idea of how the ACLS algorithms work.

www.drugs.com - This website has loads of information about pharmacology, including a pill identifier (just input the pill's physical characteristics into the database and there you go!), an interactions checker and a whole section for health professionals.

www.mayoclinic.org - I used this website a ton when researching diseases and conditions, especially when I just needed a layperson's level of knowledge or a general introduction. This comes in handy if you are creating educational materials for a patient, or just needed a very general idea of a particular disease or procedure. Most of the information I utilized was in the "patient care and health info" section of the site. The "for medical professionals" section has some nifty videos. Enjoy!

THANK YOU

Thanks again for taking time out of your busy schedule to read this book, I think you'll be thanking yourself once you see how much these tips can help you thrive in nursing school.

Please visit the website at www.straightanursingstudent.com for all the resources mentioned in this book, including:

- pre-semester checklist
- links to recommended books
- links to all the websites mentioned in Appendix B
- example of a concept map
- a variety of topics that can help you in school and on the job

See you there!

Made in the USA
Columbia, SC
20 August 2020

This book stays in my purse even though I've read it twice already. I will continue to use it as a reference throughout my program. *-Dawn*

From organization to the basics of nursing practice, this helpful book made me feel a million times better about starting my program. *-Erica*

I am so glad to have this book to help me get started with Nursing School and to help me all the way past graduation! YOU NEED THIS BOOK! *-Carlie*

A well written, information packed page turner. *-Billie*

GREAT tips in the book! I'm so prepared for school now. *-Dawn*

Study tips, organizational gems, clinical wisdom & more!

ISBN 9781500956363

90000

9 781500 956363